Personal Electronic Health Record System: Australian Perspectives

Jun Xu

King's Own Institute

Sydney, Australia

Preface

Personal electronic health records (PEHRs) (or very often called electronic health records (EHRs)) are electronic repositories of information regarding the health status of individuals, which can be managed via Internet and other electronic networks. EHRs underpin all the other e-health initiative and can play important role in enhancing the efficiency & quality of health care and reducing medical errors. A nation-wide personal electronic heath record system (i.e., the PCEHR (personally controlled electronic health record) system being implemented in Australia) has the potential to dramatically improve the patient care & health services delivery and bring huge economic benefits to Australia. However, like any large scare IS/IT projects, the PCEHR system implementation in Australia has been facing many challenges and issues, and many of them are non-technological ones. This book can be used as a good reference book for understanding the status of the implementation of the PCEHR system in Australia and challenges & issues associated with the implementation. This book also can serve as the guide book for the implementation of nation-wide personal electronic health record system in terms of suggesting factors and variables required for the successful implementation.

This book has 5 chapters. Chapter 1 discusses the background of the implementation of personal electronic health record system (i.e., PCEHR system) in Australia, it also reviews key issues & concerns associated with the implementation of the PCEHR system in Australia. In addition, this chapter also unveils relevant factors and models for examining adoption and continued use of personal electronic health record system, such factors and models will lay foundation for subsequent discussion and studies reported in the book. Chapter 2 looks at the understanding of and the current status of adoption and use of the personally controlled electronic health record (PCEHR) system among Australian consumers and Australian doctors and aims to identify concerns/issues associated with the PCEHR system and factors influencing their decision regarding adoption and use of the PCEHR system. Qualitative field studies were undertaken, in which 30 consumers/individual users and 10 doctors were interviewed. Chapter 3 discusses the development of the survey questionnaire of adoption and continued use of the PCEHR system in Australia, which includes sections of survey definitions, demographic information questions, questions on involvement in the PCEHR system, Questions on Current State of Adoption and Use of the PCEHR System, and Questions on Statements Regarding the PCEHR System. Chapter 4 presents a study of surveying consumers/individual users in Australia by applying the survey questionnaire of PCEHR system adoption and continued use discussed in Chapter 3. The results of the survey suggest that while the consumers/individual users could use the system for storing and sharing their health information, they are deeply concerned about privacy and security perspectives of their health information in the system. And the results also suggest that health care providers (e.g., doctors) have significant impact on consumers in terms of adopting and using the PCEHR system. Chapter 5 reports a study testing the model of PCERH system adoption and continued use discussed in Chapter 1. The data were collected via online questionnaire surveys and were analysed via Structural Equation Modelling (SEM) approach. Identified significant factors influencing the decision regarding system adoption include "External Factors & Influences", "Individual Differences", "Perceived Benefits" of the PCEHR system, PCEHR "System Characteristics", "Perceived User Friendliness" and "Voluntariness of Adoption", while "Realized Benefits", "Realized User Friendliness" and "Voluntariness of Continued Use" are significant factors influencing the decision regarding the continued use of the PCEHR system. The outcomes of the research lead to suggestions to assist the Australian Government in the ongoing rollout/implementation of the system.

I would like to thank Mr John Hammond, Dr Nicky Antonius, Dr Xiangzhu Gao, Dr Golam Sorwar, Dr Daniel O'Sheedy, Professor Peter Croll, and Professor Mohammed Quaddus, for their suggestions and assistance.

Jun Xu
King's Own Institute
Sydney, Australia
October 2022

Table of Contents

Chapter 1

Overview and Background of Personal Electronic Health Record System in Australia

The journey of personal electronic health record system in Australia started about 20 years ago. After the development of many stand-alone and stated-wide systems, a nation-wide system (namely Personally Controlled Electronic Health Record (PCEHR) system and it was renamed as My Health Record System later) was implemented by the Australian federal government in July 2012. The implementation of the PCEHR system in Australia has not been easy, and it has been facing many challenges and issues.

Keywords: E-health, Electronic Health Record Systems, PCEHR System, My Health Record, Australia.

1.1 Background

Electronic health records (EHRs) are electronic repositories of information regarding the health status of individuals, which can be managed via the Internet and other electronic networks. The health information includes general information (geographic, demographic, habit, family health histories,), physical or biological characteristics (height, weight, blood type), personal data (allergies and alerts, disabilities, chronic conditions, sexual health, immunisations), medical information (doctor visits, diagnoses, medications, problem lists, measurements, observations, pathology orders, imaging orders, test results, event summaries, discharge summaries, specialist letters, referrals), and other information (Medicare/veteran affairs, care plans, consumer-entered notes). EHRs underpin all the other e-health initiatives, and can assist in consumer/patient-focused approach to health information management, improvement of health service providers' ability to provide more effective and efficient services with maximized benefits to consumers/patients and minimized errors and re-admissions (Xu et al. 2013; McQuade-Jones, et al., 2014). Many countries have embarked on EHR systems, but the success of such initiatives has been low, if not very low. Studying e-health in seven countries comprising U.S., Canada, U.K., Germany, Netherlands, Australia and New Zealand, Jha et al. (2008) suggest that only those countries that are willing to put in significant investment and develop standards for medical data interchanges will realize the benefits of EHRs. In addition, large-scale government IS/IT projects (such as the nation-wide implementation of the PCEHR system) typically have large budgets and long timeframes, unfortunately they often failed because of cost overruns, time slippage, technical shortfalls, impairing performance and fail to obtain anticipated benefits (Laudon & Laudon 2014 p.560).

Much of the medical information in Australia is held in paper-based files or non-shared databases. The information may be inconsistent between files/databases, inaccurate because of lack of standards, incorrect because of manual operation, and is often not available in emergency situations (Department of Health and Aging, 2012; Xu et al., 2012). According to the Department of Health and Ageing (2012), every year an Australian had "22 interactions with healthcare providers, including 4 visits to GPs, 12 prescriptions, 3 visits to specialists". Patients may undergo the same tests with different healthcare providers. It is not unusual that the same questions are asked every time a patient visits a different provider. According to the Australian Nursing Journal (2011), Burmester (2012) and NEHTA (2012), 18% of medical errors in Australia occur from inadequate information; nearly 30% of unplanned hospital admissions are associated with prescribing errors; and approximately 13% of healthcare provider consultations suffer missing information.

Consideration of EHR systems in Australia started in 2000 (Xu et al. 2013). MediConnect, which electronically collected and stored information about medicines and exchanged such information among doctors, pharmacists and individuals, is the first system of this kind. In 2004, MediConnect completed its field test in Launceston and Ballarat and ceased as a stand-alone system on December 31, 2004. As the largest e-health trials in Australia by then, the completed field test of MediConnect provided vital experience in implementing an EHR system, and the key components of MediConnect and lessons learned from deploying the system was used to assist in the subsequent state-wide implementation of HealthConnect, which is a network of EHRs and involves electronically collecting, storing and exchanging individuals' health information on the network (Medicare 2012; Xu et al. 2013). The HealthConnect program, which started in 2005 and completed in 2009, eventually consisted of a set of different projects undertaken individually by all the states/territories except Queensland. The program provided significant gains in the establishment of e-health infrastructure across Australia (Xu et al. 2013).

In the period of 2010 to 2012, the Australian government invested $467 million in the first release of the national PCEHR system (Xu et al. 2013). Some key events leading to the first release of the national PCEHR system include: (1) the establishment of the NEHTA to coordinate the national EHR project in 2005; (2) the development of National E-health Strategy in 2008; (3) the development of the PCEHR system based on the previous initiatives of MediConnect and HealthConnect commenced in 2010; (4) the release of the Healthcare Identifiers Act 2010; (5) the pilot-testing of the PCEHR system in 12 sites across the nation in 2010; (6) The completion of Privacy Impact Assessment Report of the PCEHR system in 2011; (7) the release of Concept of Operations of the PCEHR system in 2011; (8) the announcement of the Practice Incentives Program (PIP) e-Health Incentive in 2012; (9) the release of the Personally Controlled Electronic Health Records Act 2012; and (10) the release of the PCEHR system in July 2012 (Xu et al. 2013).

The successful implementation of the PCEHR system could bring huge economic benefits to Australia. According to an estimate by international consulting firm Deloitte Consulting, the PCEHR system could generate approximately A$11.5 billion in net direct benefits over the period 2010 to 2025, with A$9.5 billion accruing to Australian governments and A$2 billion accruing to the private sector including public hospitals, GPs, specialists, allied health clinics, private hospitals and private health insurance providers (Department of Health and Aging, 2012). The Australian Government has invested significantly in deploying the PCEHR system and its associated infrastructure (e.g., more than A$1 billion since its introduction (Kerlin and Heath, 2014), and in its 2017-2018 Budget, a further A$374.2 million over the next two years (Australian Government, 2017), but the system has not been well received by consumers and health care providers.

The Australian Government invested A$467 million in the personally controlled electronic health record (PCEHR) (recently rebadged as My Health Record) system during the period 2010 to 2012 (NEHTA, 2011). This PCEHR system allows doctors, hospitals and other healthcare providers to share individuals' health information in order to provide the best possible medical care

(Department of Health 2016). The first version of the PCEHR system was released on 1 July 2012, when Australian residents were invited to register online (i.e., opt-in approach). In 2012, the Australian Government committed an additional A$233.7 million for deploying and refining the PCEHR system, and a further A$485 million in 2015 (Department of Health, 2015). In its 2017-2018 Budget, further A$374.2 million over next two years were allocated for the PCEHR (Australian Government 2017). After the low participation rate of initial opt-in approach, the Australian government considers an opt-out approach (Department of Health 2015), and trials of opt-out approach were conducted in 2016 (Coyne, 2016). In 2018, the opt-out approach is enforced, and individuals can opt out by 15 October 2018, and the opt-out due date was later changed to 31 January 2019 (My Health Record, 2018).

The PCEHR (renamed My Health Record) system is far from mature and suffers criticisms from major stakeholders, and there is a lack of uptake and utilization (Partel, 2015). For example, Xu et al. (2013) point out the following concerns and issues which could have impact on the delivery, management and success of the PCEHR system:

- Uncertainty of the government (e.g., the change of federal and state government every 3-4 years)
- Uncertainty of the economy (e.g., the unstable commodity market)
- Difficulties of achieving a unified approach (e.g., Australia's multi-tier government has made the implementation of the PCEHR system extremely complex and challenging)
- The lack of transparency and communication of the PCEHR system implementation from government agencies.
- The Australian Government's initial choice of opt-in approach, which was later changed to opt-out approach as a result of very low adoption rate.
- Privacy concerns (e.g., consumers were not certain about and had no confidence in the privacy protection measures provided by the system and no clear communications regarding such issues were provided)
- Effectiveness and Usability issues of the PCEHR system (e.g., it went live in July 2012 with more than 60 high security and critical bugs without proper back-up and disaster recovery measures. And It was argued that the PCEHR system was not properly tested before its release. Meanwhile, the interoperability of the PCEHR system with many existing systems of health care providers was another significant challenge).

The interests of consumers have not been properly represented in the development and implementation of the PCEHR system. In the PCEHR review ordered by the Coalition Government, no review panel members represented consumers. The initial policy for adoption of the system is based on an opt-in approach, but users are not enthusiastic in registering with and using the system (Sansom, 2016; Swinn and Weber, 2017) for different reasons and various concerns. The Australian Government considers an opt-out approach (Department of Health, 2015), and trials of the opt-out approach were conducted in 2016 (Coyne, 2016). In 2018, the opt-out approach is enforced, and individuals can opt out initially by 31 January 2019 (My Health Record, 2018). The existing concerns about privacy, security and system operation and wrong perceptions of the benefits would be the main reason for the opt-out of the system (Gribbin, 2018; Grubb, 2018; McCauley, 2018; Minion, 2018; Murphy, 2018). In addition, the long-term and sustainable success of the system requires far more resources and efforts beyond the initial registration stage.

Even though the Australian government has invested significantly in deploying the system and its associated infrastructure (including required technological infrastructure, standards, legislations, and others), but the system has not been well received by consumers/patients and health care providers. In addition, there is a lack of the comprehensive empirical studies of the current status and challenges/issues as well as the reasons and factors for success and failure of electronic health record systems, especially PCEHR (My Health Record).

1.2 A Research Model of Adoption and Continued Use of Personal Electronic Personal Health Record System

1.2.1 Underlining Models

Xu, Gao and Sorwar (2014) model of consumers' adoption and continued use of the PCEHR system, developed from Xu and Quaddus (2007) model of Adoption and Continued Use of Knowledge Management Systems (KMSs) (see Figure-1), is adopted to examine the adoption and continued use of the PCEHR system in Australia. Xu and Quaddus (2007) model is built on the theory of diffusion of innovations (Rogers 1995), theory of reasoned action (TRA) (Ajzen & Fishbein 1980), and technology acceptance model (TAM) (Davis 1986). These three theories are the primary theoretical foundations for many research projects on IT acceptance and use. While theory of diffusion of innovations focuses on the diffusion process of an innovation, TRA and TAM models attempt to explain the relationship between user attitudes, perceptions, beliefs, and actual use of a technology. Basically, their model suggests that some external factors influence the perceptions about a knowledge management system, which in turn affect the adoption of the innovation and lead to the use of the system, i.e. "External Factors" >> "Views & Perceptions" >> "Adoption Decision" (for pre-adoption stage) "Facilitating Condition/External Factors" >> Realization of Benefits & Consequences" >> "Continued Use" (for post-adoption stage). This simple model is generic in nature and is likely to be applicable, with some adjustments, in various innovation diffusion processes. This simple research model also serves as the conceptual framework for the development of the PCEHR adoption and continued use model.

Xu and Quaddus's (2007) pre and post adoption model of KMS is unique, and is different from other IS adoption/diffusion models, which only deal with either pre-adoption stage or post-adoption stage. In the pre-adoption stage, it suggests that external influences, including individual difference factors, organisational factors, task complexity factors, organic factors, will influence the adoption of knowledge management systems in an indirect way with their influence being mediated by the perceived benefits (usefulness) and perceived user friendliness (ease of use) of KMSs (Rogers 1995; Davis 1986; Davis, Bagozzi and Warshaw 1989; Ajzen and Fishbein 1980; Moore 1987; Agarwal and Prasad 1999; Liker and Sindi 1997; Igbaria 1994; Igbaria, Guimaraes and Davis 1995; Igbaria et al. 1997). At the same time, the research model postulates that the perceived factors of perceived benefits, perceived user-friendliness (ease of use), subject norms (i.e., influence from people who are important to the user (Ajzen and Fishbein 1980)), and perceived voluntariness (i.e., the degree of voluntary use (Moore and Benbasat 1991) have direct effect on the adoption of KMSs. Also as per TAM (Davis 1986, 1989, 1993; Davis, Bagozzi and Warshaw 1989), perceived user friendliness affects perceived usefulness. In the post-adoption stage, it is suggested that organizational facilitation factors will influence the continued use of knowledge management systems in an indirect way with their influence being mediated by the realized benefits (usefulness) and realized user friendliness (ease of use) of KMSs (Rogers 1995; Davis 1986; Davis, Bagozzi and Warshaw 1989; Ajzen and Fishbein 1980; Moore 1987; Agarwal and Prasad 1999; Liker and Sindi 1997; Igbaria 1994; Igbaria, Guimaraes and Davis 1995; Igbaria et al. 1997). At the same time, the research model postulates that the perceived factors of perceived benefits, perceived user-friendliness (ease of use), subject norms, and perceived voluntariness have direct effect on the continued use of KMSs. Also as per TAM (Davis 1986, 1989, 1993; Davis, Bagozzi and Warshaw 1989), perceived user friendliness affects perceived usefulness.

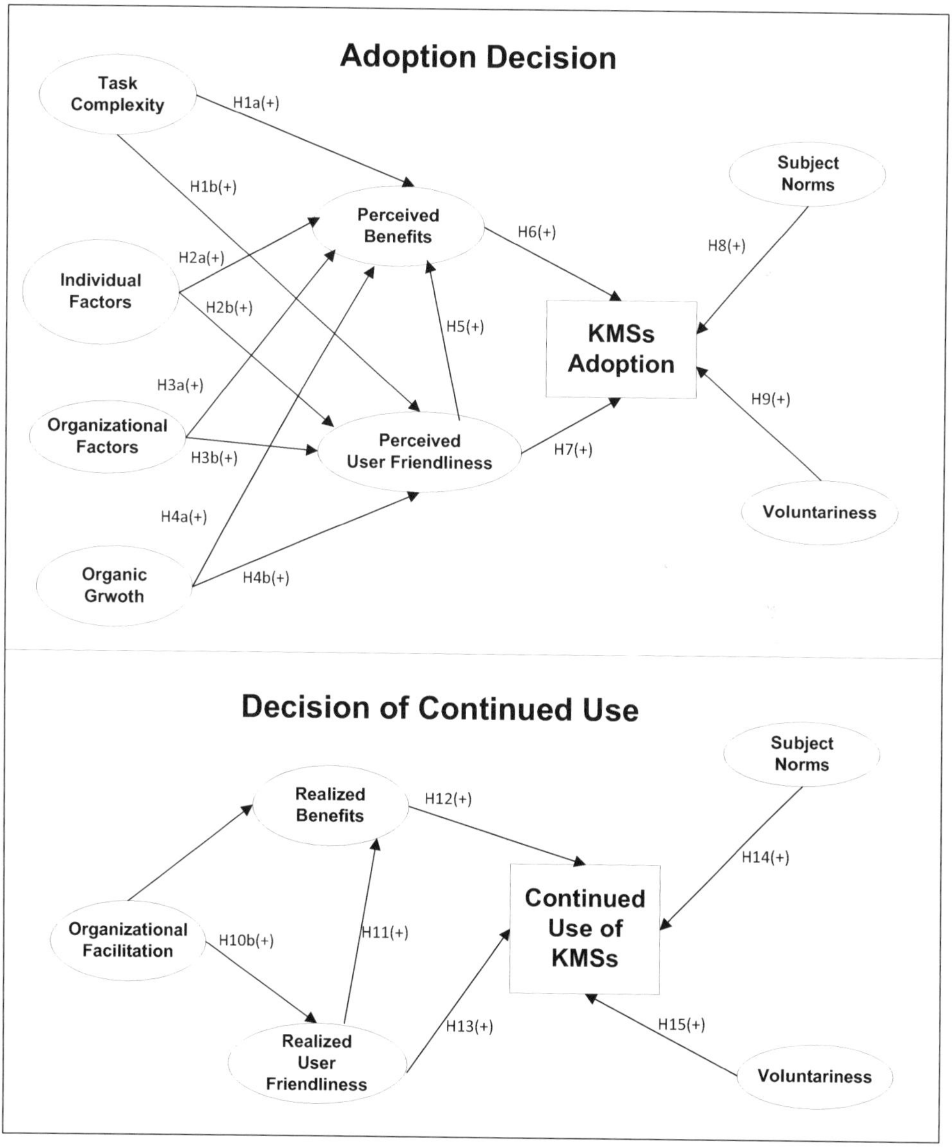

Figure-1: Xu & Quaddus's (2007) model of adoption and continued use of KMSs

Using Xu and Quaddus' (2007) model as the basis, Xu, Gao and Sorwar (2014) develop a research model of adoption and continued use of PCEHR system. The research model (see Figure-2) includes two parts: (1) pre-adoption stage and post-adoption stage (see Figure-2). The proposed pre and post adoption model of PCEHR system is unique, and is different from other IS/IT adoption/diffusion models, which only deal with either pre-adoption stage or post-adoption stage. In the pre-adoption stage, it suggests that the external factors including external environment & influences, individual differences, and PCEHR system characteristics will influence the adoption of the PCEHR systems in an indirect way with their influence being mediated by the perceived benefits (usefulness) and perceived user friendliness (ease of use) of the system. At the same time, the research model postulates that the factors of perceived benefits, perceived user-friendliness (ease of use), subject norms, and perceived voluntariness have direct effect on the adoption of the PCEHR system, and it also indicates that perceived user friendliness affects perceived usefulness.

In the post-adoption stage, it is suggested that the organizational facilitation factors will influence the continued use of the PCEHR system in an indirect way with their influence being mediated by the realized benefits(usefulness) and realized user friendliness (ease of use) of the system, and it also suggests that realized user friendliness affects realized benefits (Rogers 1995; Davis 1986; Davis, Bagozzi & Warshaw 1989; Ajzen & Fishbein 1980; Moore 1987; Agarwal & Prasad 1999; Liker & Sindi 1997; Igbaria 1994; Igbaria, Guimaraes & Davis 1995; Igbaria et al. 1997).

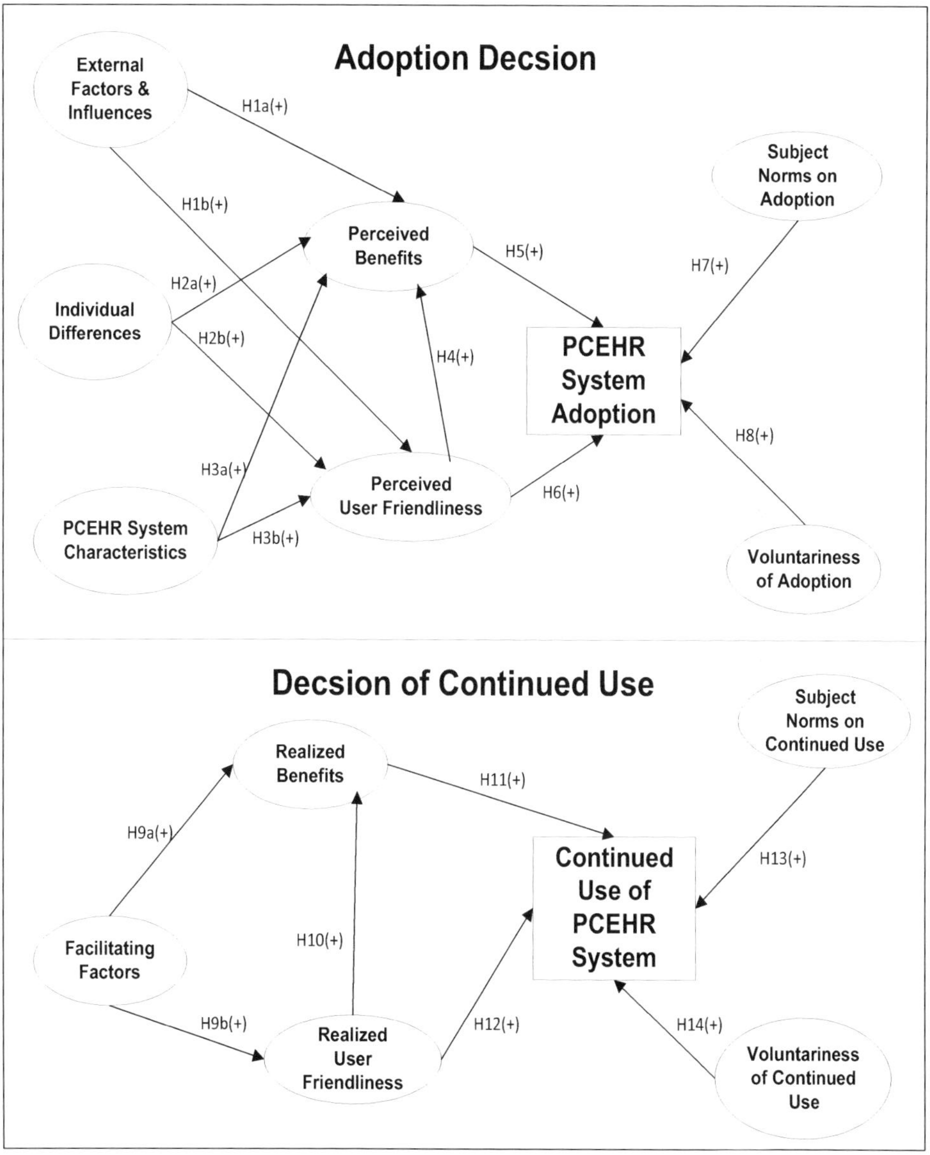

Figure-2: The Research Model (Source: Xu, Gao & Sorwar 2014)

1.2.2 Hypotheses Development

Past studies (Grover, 1993; Premkumar et al., 1997; Rai and Bajwa, 1997; Sarvary, 1999; Xu and Quaddus, 2009; Xu et al., 2012; Xu et al., 2013; Xu et al., 2014) report environmental factors are associated with adoption of innovation. In addition, Davis' (1986) technology acceptance model proposes that external factors, such as external factors and influences, will influence PCEHR system adoption by affecting perceived benefits and perceived user friendliness. Some perspectives of External Factors and Influences include: Regulations and policies relevant to the PCEHR system (e.g., Healthcare Identifiers Act 2010; Personally Controlled Electronic Health Records Act 2012; My Health Records Act 2012), deployment and investment in e-health ICT infrastructure, the increasing mobility of population, the wide availability of computing equipment and the huge popularity of mobile devices, affordability and accessibility of internet services, the uncertainty of the Australian economy, the continuity of government, Australia's multi-tier government system and large private sector, and poor transparency and lack of communication regarding the operations of the responsible agency (e.g., former National E-health Transition Authority (NEHTA)) and information regarding the implementation of the PCEHR system (Anderson, 2007; Xu and Quaddus, 2007; Xu and Quaddus, 2009; Vest, 2010; Xu and Quaddus, 2012; Xu et al., 2012; Xu et al., 2013; Pearce and Bainbridge, 2014; Xu et al., 2014; Partel, 2015; Cohen, 2016; Eden et al., 2016; Jawhari et al., 2016; Sherer et al., 2016; Brinkel et al., 2017).

The preceding discussion leads to the following hypothesis:

Hypothesis 1a: "External Factors & Influences" positively influence the "Perceived Benefits" of the PCEHR System.

Hypothesis 1b: "External Factors & Influences" positively influence the "Perceived User Friendliness" of the PCEHR System.

Individual differences have been found important in explaining the acceptance and successful implementation of information systems (Igbaria et al., 1995). Past research (Zmud, 1979; Brancheau and Wetherbe, 1990; Rogers, 1995; Gefen and Straub, 1997; Agarwal and Prasad, 1999; Agarwal and Prasad, 2000; Venkatesh and Davis, 2000; Xu and Quaddus, 2007; Aggelidis and Chatzoglou, 2009; Xu and Quaddus, 2009; Xu et al., 2012; Xu et al., 2013) has indicated that the individual/end user characteristics/differences are important factors in explaining/predicting the adoption of innovations. In addition, Davis' (1986) technology acceptance model (TAM) proposes that external factors, such as individual factors, will influence PCEHR system adoption by affecting perceived benefits and perceived user friendliness. The PCEHR system is only successful if the users of the system persist with the system. Australian consumers' acceptance and use of the system is critical to the success of the system. Some perspectives of Individual Differences/Factors include: Involvement in the deployment of the PCEHR system, experience/skill in using new systems and new technologies, willingness to try new systems and new technologies (e.g., the PCEHR system), age, education level, occupation/profession, income level, family composition, location, and attitude toward managing medical information electronically (Xu and Quaddus, 2007; Ludwick and Doucette, 2009; Xu and Quaddus, 2009; Xu and Quaddus, 2012; Xu et al., 2012; Xu et al., 2013; Nguyen et al., 2014; Xu et al., 2014; Sligo et al., 2017) .

Hence, it is hypothesised that:

Hypothesis 2a: "Individual factors" positively influence the "Perceived Benefits" of the PCEHR system.

Hypothesis 2b: "Individual factors" positively influence the "Perceived User Friendliness" of the PCEHR system.

Past studies (Kwon and Zmud, 1987; Moore, 1987; Davis et al., 1992; Igbaria et al., 1995; Rogers, 1995; Agarwal and Prasad, 1997; Chau and Tam, 1997; Beatty et al., 2001; Hong et al., 2002; Xu and Quaddus, 2007; Xu and Quaddus, 2009; Xu and Quaddus, 2012; Xu et al., 2013) indicate the importance of the innovation/system characteristics in the adoption and diffusion of innovation. In addition, Davis' (1986) technology acceptance model (TAM) proposes that external factors, such as PCEHR system characteristics, will influence adoption of the system by affecting perceived benefits and perceived user friendliness. Some perspectives of the PCEHR System Characteristics include: trialability of the PCEHR system, accuracy, completeness, and currency of information in the system, visibility and transparency of the system, information control, children medical information management, accessibility, availability, regional/district integration of applications and systems of various health care providers, cross-state integration of applications and systems of various health care providers, international integration of applications and systems of various health care providers, regular maintenances and updates, and delegation options (Xu and Quaddus, 2007; Ludwick and Doucette 2009; Xu and Quaddus, 2009; Xu and Quaddus, 2012; Xu et al., 2012; Xu et al., 2013; Jamoom et al., 2014; Kerai et al., 2014; Nguyen et al., 2014; Pearce and Bainbridge, 2014; Thurston, 2014; Xu et al., 2014; ; Partel, 2015; Barbarin et al., 2016; Chao, 2016; Eden et al., 2016;

Jawhari et al. 2016; Palojoki et al., 2016; Sansom, 2016; Cunningham et al., 2017; Sligo et al., 2017; Swinn and Weber, 2017).

The above discussion lead to the following hypothesis:

Hypothesis 3a: "PCEHR System Characteristics" positively influence the "Perceived Benefits" of the PCEHR System.

Hypothesis 3b: PCEHR System Characteristics" positively influence the "Perceived User Friendliness" of the PCEHR System.

TAM (Davis, 1986, 1989, 1993; Davis et al., 1989) and other related studies (Adams et al., 1992; Igbaria et al., 1995; Igbaria et al., 1997; Venkatesh and Davis, 2000; Xu and Quaddus, 2007; Aggelidis and Chatzoglou, 2009; Holden and Karsh, 2010) have identified perceived user friendliness as an important determinant of system acceptance and use via perceived benefits and a causal determinant of perceived benefits. Perceived user friendliness has a direct and positive impact on perceived benefits. Some perspectives of User Friendliness (and Realized User Friendliness) include: Simple to learn and use the system, cheap to learn and use the system, fast to retrieve the required information in the system, privacy and security measures, human assistance and interaction opportunities while using the system, multi-channels and multiple touch points of accessing the system, and opportunities to network with users of the system (Anderson, 2007; Xu and Quaddus, 2007; Xu and Quaddus, 2009; Xu and Quaddus, 2012; Xu et al., 2012; Xu et al., 2013; Nguyen et al., 2014; Xu et al., 2014; Partel, 2015; Asan et al., 2016; Barbarin et al., 2016; Eden et al., 2016; Jawhari et al., 2016; Brinkel et al., 2017; Hoque and Sorwar, 2017; Swinn and Weber, 2017); and some perspectives of benefits (and realized benefits) of the PCEHR system include: Personal medical information management, better and new services, efficiency/productivity, effectiveness, quality, safety, time and cost reduction, continuity of health services, health/well-being, saving lives, and equitable access to health services (Xu and Quaddus, 2007; Xu and Quaddus, 2009; Xu and Quaddus, 2012; Xu et al., 2012; Xu et al., 2013; Jamoom et al., 2014; Nguyen et al., 2014; Thurston, 2014; Xu et al., 2014; Asan et al., 2016; Chao, 2016; Brinkel et al., 2017; Hoque and Sorwar, 2017; Swinn and Weber, 2017).

Therefore, the following hypotheses are proposed:

Hypothesis 4: "Perceived User Friendliness" of PCEHR System positively influences the "Perceived Benefits" of the PCEHR System.

Hypothesis 10: "Realized User Friendliness" of PCEHR System positively influences the "Realized Benefits" of the PCEHR System.

The theory of diffusion of innovation (Rogers, 1995), the theory of reasoned action (Ajzen and Fishbein, 1978), and the technology acceptance model (Davis, 1986) all propose direct impacts of perceptions on intention to use the system. Past research (Bansler and Havn, 2002; Aggelidis and Chatzoglou, 2009; Holden and Karsh, 2010; Martins et al., 2014) suggest that expectations/perceptions are significant factors in determining users' adoption decision of an information system, and that users' confirmation of their initial use of information systems has a positive impact on their intention of continued use of the system (Bhattacherjee, 2001). As a result, it is proposed that perceived benefits and perceived user friendliness have a direct impact on PCEHR system adoption and continued use (i.e., for uploading and storing medical information into the PCEHR system, disseminating and sharing medical information with various health service providers and government agencies via the PCEHR system, and using the PCEHR system to manage medical information (Xu and Quaddus, 2007; Xu and Quaddus, 2009; Xu and Quaddus, 2012; Xu et al., 2012; Xu et al., 2013; Jamoom et al., 2014; Nguyen et al., 2014; Xu et al., 2014).

As per the above discussion, it is hypothesised that:

Hypothesis 5: "Perceived Benefits" of PCEHR System positively influence the "Adoption" of the PCEHR System.

Hypothesis 6: "Perceived User Friendliness" of PCEHR System positively influence the "Adoption" of the PCEHR System.

Hypothesis 11: "Realized Benefits" of PCEHR System positively influence the "Continued Use" of the PCEHR System.

Hypothesis 12: "Realized User Friendliness" of PCEHR System positively influence the "Continued Use" of the PCEHR System.

Subject Norms describe the social influence that may affect a person's intention to use the PCEHR system. People often take action based on their perceptions of what others think they should do. Literature (Thompson et al., 1991; Liker and Sindi, 1997; Lucas and Spitler, 1999, Xu and Quaddus, 2007; Aggelidis and Chatzoglou, 2009; Holden and Karsh, 2010) has found that subject norms are positively associated with individual's acceptance of new technology. For the acceptance and use of the PCERH system, doctors and health service providers can exert considerable influence (Cowan, 2016; Sansom, 2016; Swinn and Weber, 2017). Meanwhile, Gray (2000) suggests that use of an information system (i.e., knowledge management system) may be a self-reinforcing process. Once the value of such a system is established, the system use is likely to become routine and thus lead to widespread acceptance and use. Some perspectives of Subject Norms include: Peer pressure/influence, following earlier users' lead, respected people's influence, doctor's recommendation, and media influence (Xu and Quaddus, 2007; Xu and Quaddus, 2009; Xu and Quaddus, 2012; Xu et al., 2012; Xu et al., 2013; Xu et al., 2014; Asan et al., 2016; Brinkel et al., 2017; Hoque and Sorwar, 2017).

The above discussion results in the following hypotheses:

Hypothesis 7: "Subject Norms" positively influence the "Adoption" of the PCEHR System.

Hypothesis 13: "Subject Norms" positively influence the "Continued Use" of the PCEHR System.

Voluntariness focuses on consumers' voluntary adoption and use of the PCEHR system. Past research (Bansler and Havn, 2002; Xu and Quaddus, 2007; Xu et al., 2014) has suggested that a voluntary-basis approach has a positive impact on people's decisions to adopt and use innovations/new systems. The opt-in model has not been working well, and it is argued that the opt-out model could increase the adoption rate of the PCEHR system (Pearce and Bainbridge, 2014; Partel, 2015; Coyne, 2017; Cunningham et al., 2017; Swinn and Weber, 2017). However the privacy and security concerns as well as the mishandling and mismanagement of the implementation of the current system could encourage individuals to opt-out of the system and create wrong perceptions about the benefits of the system (Gribbin, 2018; Grubb, 2018; McCauley, 2018; Minion, 2018; Murphy, 2018). The opt-out approach could increase the (mandatory) uptake of the system, but individual users would still prefer to have the option and be given the opportunity to make their own decisions. In addition, forced initial uptake and use of the system may not lead to the subsequent continued use of the system since the users would make their decisions of continued use based on their experiences and realized benefits (Agarwal and Prasad, 1997).

The above discussions lead to the following hypotheses:

Hypothesis 8: "Voluntary use" of PCEHR System positively influences the "Adoption" of the PCEHR System.

Hypothesis 14: "Voluntary use" of PCEHR System positively influences the "Continued Use" of the PCEHR System.

Governments face the challenge of how to ensure consumers' sustained use of the PCEHR system after their adoption of the system. Sustained/continued use of the PCEHR system means that use of the system has become a part of consumers' everyday life. By providing facilitating measures (such as incentives, imperatives, policy updates, system improvements, promotion of success stories and best practices, promotion of benefits, satisfying consumers' needs, and making use of the PCEHR system a part of the user's life), governments could modify consumers' positive attitudes to and perceptions of the system and thus lead to their continued use of the system. In addition, the literature (Ajzen and Fishbein, 1978; Rogers, 1985; Davis, 1986; Holden and Karsh, 2010) all propose direct impacts of perceptions on intention to use an information system. Some perspectives of Facilitating Factors include: Incentives, imperatives, policy updates, system improvements, promotion of success stories and best practices, promotion of benefits, satisfying consumers' needs, and making use of the PCEHR system a part of the user's everyday life (Anderson, 2007; Xu and Quaddus, 2007; Aggelidis and Chatzoglou, 2009; Xu and Quaddus, 2009; Xu and Quaddus, 2012; Xu et al., 2012; Xu et al., 2013; Jamoom et al., 2014; Pearce and Bainbridge, 2014; Xu et al., 2014; Partel, 2015; Cohen, 2016; Jawhari et al., 2016; Sansom, 2016; Sherer et al., 2016; Sligo et al., 2017; Swinn and Weber, 2017). As a result, it is proposed that perceived benefits and perceived user friendliness have a direct impact on continued use of PCEHR system.

The above discussion results in the following hypotheses:

Hypothesis 9a: "Facilitating Factors" positively influence the "Realized Benefits" of the PCEHR System.

Hypothesis 9b: "Facilitating Factors" positively influence the "Realized User Friendliness" of the PCEHR System.

1.3 Summary

This chapter discusses the background of the implementation of personal electronic health record system (i.e., PCEHR system) in Australia, it also reviews key issues & concerns associated with the implementation of the PCEHR system in Australia. In addition, this chapter also unveils relevant factors and models for examining adoption and continued use of personal electronic health record system, such factors and models will lay foundation for subsequent discussion and studies reported in the book.

Acknowledgement
This chapter is developed from the author's previous works: (1) "Implementation of E-Health Record Systems in Australia", *International Technology Management Review*, 2013, Vol. 3, No.2, pp. 92-104; (2) "A research model of consumers' adoption and continued use of the Personally Controlled Electronic Health Record (PCEHR) system", *International Technology Management Review*, 2014, Vol. 4, No.4, pp. 187-200.

References

Agarwal, R. and Prasad, J. (1997), "The Role of Innovation Characteristics and Perceived Voluntariness in the Acceptance of Information Technologies", Decision Sciences, Vol. 28, No. 3, pp. 557-582.

Agarwal, R. and Prasad, J. (1999), "Are Individual Differences Germane to the Acceptance of New Information Technologies", Decision Sciences, Vol. 30, No. 2, pp. 361-391.

Agarwal , R. and Prasad, J. (2000), "A field study of the adoption of software process innovations by information systems professionals", IEEE Transaction on Engineering Management, Vol. 47, No. 3, pp. 295-308.

Aggelidis, V. P. and Chatzoglou, P. D. (2009), "Using a modified technology acceptance model in hospitals", International Journal of Medical Informatics, Vol. 78, pp.115-126.

Ajzen, I. and Fishbein, M. (1980), Understanding Attitudes and Predicting Social Behavior, Prentice-Hall, Inc., Englewood Cliffs, New Jersey 07632.

Anderson, J. G. (2007), "Social, ethical and legal barriers to E-health", International Journal of Medical Informatics, Vol. 76, pp.480-483.

Australian Government (2017), Budget 2017-2018: Budget Statements 2017-18 Budget Related Paper No. 1.10, Health Portfolio, Online Available at: http://www.health.gov.au/internet/budget/publishing.nsf/Content/2017-2018_Health_PBS_sup4/$File/2017-18_Health_PBS_Complete.pdf (accessed on 14 May 2017).

Australian Nursing Journal, (2011), "News: National E-health rollout on", Australian Nursing Journal, Vol. 18, No. 10, p.5.

Barbarin, A. M., Klasnja, P. and Veinot, T. C. (2016), "Good or bad, ups and downs, and getting better: Use of personal health data for temporal reflection in chronic illness", International Journal of Medical Informatics, Vol. 94, pp. 237-245.

Beatty, R.C., Shim, J. P., and Jones, M.C. (2001), "Factors influencing corporate website adoption: a time-based assessment", Information & Management, Vol. 38, No. 6, pp. 337-354.

Bentler, P. M. and Chou, C. P. (1987), "Practical issues in Structural Modelling", Sociological Methods & Research, Vol. 16, No. 1, pp.78-117.

Bhattacherjee, A. (2001), "Understanding Information Systems Continuance: An Expectation-Confirmation Model", MIS Quarterly, Vol. 25, No. 3, pp. 351-370.

Brancheau, J. C. and Wetherbe, J. C. (1990), "The adoption of spreadsheet software: testing innovation diffusion theory in the context of end-user computing", Information Systems Research, Vol. 1, No. 2, pp. 123-139.

Brinkel, J., Dako-Gyeke, P., Kramer, A., May, J. and Fobil, J. N. (2017), "An investigation of user attitudes, requirements and willingness to use mobile phone-based interactive voice response systems for seeking healthcare in Ghana: A qualitative study", Public Health, Vol. 144, pp.125-133.

Burmester, S. (2012), Review the Progress of eHealth in Australia, Presentation by National E-Health Transition Authority, 20/03/2012.

Chao, C. A. (2016), "The impact of electronic health records on collaborative work routines: A narrative network analysis", International Journal of Medical Informatics, Vol. 94, pp.100-111.

Chau, P. Y. K. and Tam, K. Y. (1997), "Factors affecting the adoption of open systems: An exploratory study", MIS Quarterly, Vol. 21, No. 1, pp. 1-24.

Cohen, M. F. (2016), "Impacts of the HIETH financial incentives on EHR adoption in small, physician-owned practices", International Journal of Medical Informatics, Vo. 94, pp.143-154.

Coyne, A. (2016), "Australia's first opt-out e-health site to start trials this week", itnews, January 27 2016, Online Available at: http://www.itnews.com.au/news/australias-first-opt-out-ehealth-site-to-start-trials-this-week-414099 (accessed on February 22, 2016).

Coyne, A. (2017), "Budget 2017: Policy change backed by funding injection", itnews, 9 May 2017, Online Available at: https://www.itnews.com.au/news/every-australian-will-now-get-an-automatic-e-health-record-461072 (accessed on 9 May 2017).

Davis, F. D. (1986), A technology Acceptance Model for Empirically Testing New End-User Information Systems: Theory and Results, Doctoral Dissertation, Massachusetts Institute of Technology.

Davis, F. D. (1986), A technology Acceptance Model for Empirically Testing New End-User Information Systems: Theory and Results, Doctoral Dissertation, Massachusetts Institute of Technology.

Davis, F. D., Bagozzi, R. P. and Warshaw, P. R. (1989), "User acceptance of computer technology: a comparison of two theoretical models", Management Science, Vol. 35, No. 8, pp. 982-1002.

Davis, F. D., Bagozzi, R. P. and Warshaw, P. R. (1992), "Extrinsic and intrinsic motivation to use computers in the workplace", Journal of Applied Social Psychology, Vol. 22, No. 14, pp. 1111-1132.

Department of Health (2015), Patients to get new myHealth Record: $485m 'rescue' package to reboot Labor's e-health failures, Media Release, May 10, 2015, Online Available at: https://www.health.gov.au/internet/ministers/publishing.nsf/Content/health-mediarel-yr2015-ley050.htm (accessed on February 18, 2016).

Department of Health and Aging (2012), Expected Benefits of the National PCEHR System, May 2012.Dwinnell, W. (2010), Principal Components Analysis. Available: http://matlabdatamining.blogspot.com.au/2010/02/principal-components-analysis.html [Accessed 8 July 2014].

Eden, K.B., Totten, A. M., Kassakian, S. Z., Gorman, P. N., McDonagh, M.S., Devine, B., Pappas, M., Daeges, M., Woods, S. and Hersh, W. R. (2016), "Barriers and facilitators to exchanging health information: A systematic review", International Journal of Medical Informatics, Vol. 88. pp. 44-51.

Gefen, D. and Straub, D. W. (1997), "Gender differences in the perceptions and use of E-mail: an extension to the technology acceptance model", MIS Quarterly, Vol. 21, No. 4, pp. 389-400.

Gribbin, C. (2018), "My Health Record: Greg Hunt bows to pressure, announces changes to address privacy concerns", ABC News, 1 August 2018, Online, Available at: http://www.abc.net.au/news/2018-07-31/court-order-needed-for-my-health-record-greg-hunt-says/10058544 (accessed on 1 August 2018).

Grubb, B. (2018), "Australians are 'rightly' questioning My Health Record, says Privacy Commissioner", The Sydney Morning Herald, 31 July 2018, Online, Available at: https://www.smh.com.au/technology/australians-are-rightly-questioning-my-health-record-says-privacy-commissioner-20180730-p4zui3.html (accessed on 1 August 2018).

Hong, W.Y., Thong, J. Y. L., Wong, W.W. and Tam, K. Y. (2002), "Determinants of user acceptance of digital libraries: an empirical examination of individual differences and system characteristics", Journal of Management Information Systems, Vol. 18, No. 3, pp. 97-124.

Hoque, R. & Sorwar, G. (2017), "Understanding factors influencing the adoption of mHealth by the elderly: An extension of the UTAUT model", International Journal of Medical Informatics, Vol. 101, pp.75-84.

Igbaria, M. (1994), "An examination of the factors contributing to microcomputer technology acceptance", Accounting, Management & Information Technology, Vol. 4, No. 4, pp. 205-224.

Igbaria, M., Guimaraes, T. and Davis, G.B. (1995), "Testing the determinants of microcomputer usage via a structural equation model", Journal of Management Information Systems, Vol. 11, No. 4, pp. 87-114.

Igbaria, M., Zinatelli, N., Cargg, P. and Cavaye, A. L. M. (1997), "Personal Computing Acceptance Factors in Small Firms: A Structural Equation Model", MIS Quarterly, Vol. 21, No. 3, pp. 279-302.

Jamoom, E. W., Patel, V., Furukawa, M. F. and King, J. (2014), "EHR adopters vs non-adopters: Impacts of, barriers to, and federal initiatives for EHR adoption", Healthcare, Vol. 2, pp. 33-39.

Jawhari, B., Keenan, L., Zakus, D., Ludwick, D., Isaac, A., Saleh, A. and Hayward, R. (2016), "Barriers and facilitators to Electronic Medical Record (EMR) use in an urban slum", International Journal of Medical Informatics, Vol. 94, pp.246-254.

Jha, A. K., Doolan, D., Grandt, D., Scott, T. & Bates, D. W. (2008), "The use of health information technology in seven nations", International Journal of Medical Information, Vol. 77, pp.848-854.

Kerai, P., Wood, P. and Martin, M. (2014), "A pilot study on the views of elderly regional Australians of personally controlled electronic health records", International Journal of Medical Informatics, Vol. 83, pp. 201-209.

Kerlin, J. and Heath, J. (2014), "E-health scheme to be revived after panel review", The Australian Financial Review, May 24 2014, Online Available at: http://www.afr.com/business/health/pharmaceuticals/ehealth-scheme-to-be-revived-after-panel-review-20140523-iupi8 (accessed on February 18, 2016).

Kwon, T. H. and Zmud, R. W. (1987), "Unifying the fragment models of information systems implementation" in Critical Issues in Information System Research, eds R. J. Boland Jr. & R. A. Hirscheim, John Wiley & Sons, New York, pp. 227-251.

Laudon. K.C. & Laudon, J. P. (2014), Management Information Systems: Managing the Digital Firm, Thirteenth Edition, UK.

Liker, J. K. and Sindi, A. A. (1997), "User acceptance of expert systems: A test of the theory of reasoned action", Journal of Engineering and Technology Management, Vol. 14, No. 2, pp. 147-173.

Ludwick, D. A. and Doucette, J. (2009), "Adopting electronic medical records in primary care:

Lessons learned from health information systems implementation experience in seven countries", International Journal of Medical Informatics, Vol. 78, pp.22-31.

McCauley, D. (2018), "Health Minister backs down on My Health Record", The Sydney Morning Herald, 31 July 2018, Online, Available at: https://www.smh.com.au/politics/federal/health-minister-backs-down-on-my-health-record-20180731-p4zuqo.html (accessed on 1 August 2018).

McQuade-Jones, B., Murphy, J. Novak, T. and Lisa-Nicole, S. (2014), "Nurse Practitioners and Meaningful Use: Transforming Health Care", The Journal of Nursing Practitioners, Vol.10, Issue 10, pp.763-768.

Medicare, MediConnect (2012), Online available at http://www.medicareaustralia.gov.au/provider/patients/mediconnect.jsp (accessed Sep 27, 2012).

Minion, L. (2018), "Queensland threatens to disrupt My Health Record roll out with call for COAG to suspend opt out", Healthcare IT, 30 July 2018, Online, Available at: https://www.healthcareit.com.au/article/queensland-threatens-disrupt-my-health-record-roll-out-call-coag-suspend-opt-out (accessed on 1 August 2018).

Moore, G. C. (1987), "End-user computing and office automation: a diffusion of innovation perspectives', INFOR, Vol. 25, No. 3, pp. 214-235.

Murphy, K. (2018), "My Health Record: Greg Hunt promises to redraft legislation after public outcry", The Guardian, 31 July 2018, Online, Available at: https://www.theguardian.com/australia-news/2018/jul/31/my-health-record-greg-hunt-promises-to-redraft-legislation-after-public-outcry (accessed on 1 August 2018).

My Health Record (2018), Opt out of My Health Record, Online, Available at: https://www.myhealthrecord.gov.au/for-you-your-family/opt-out-my-health-record (Accessed on 9 August 2018).

NEHTA (2012), Overview of the National eHealth Strategy and the Personally Controlled Electronic Health Record, May 2012.

Partel, K. (2015), "Toward better implementation: Australia's My Health Record", Deeble Institute Issues Brief, No. 13, 30/10/2015,pp.1-20.

Pearce, C. and Bainbridge, M. (2014), "A personally controlled electronic health record for Australia", Journal of the American Medical Informatics Association, Vol. 21, pp.707-713.

Rai, A. and Bajwa, D. (1997), "An empirical investigation into factors relating to the adoption of executive information systems: an analysis of EIS for collaboration and decision support", Decisions Sciences, Vol. 28, No. 4, pp. 939-974.

Rogers, E. M. (1995), Diffusion of Innovations, Fourth Edition, The Free Press, New York, USA.

Sansom, M. (2016), "My Health Record: Medics speak up", Government News, 15 August 2016, Online Available at: http://www.governmentnews.com.au/2016/08/24703/ (accessed on 15 April 2017).

Sarvary, M. (1999), "Knowledge Management and Competition in the Consulting Industry", California Management Review, Vol. 41, No.2, pp.95-107.

Sherer, S. A., Meyerhoefer, C. D. and Peng, L. (2016), "Applying institutional theory to the adoption of electronic health records in the U.S.", Information & Management, Vol. 53, pp.570-580.

Sligo, J., Gauld, R., Roberts, V. and Villa, L. (2017), "A literature review for large-scale health information system project planning, implementation and evaluation", International Journal of Medical Informatics, Vol. 97, pp.86-97.

Swinn, M. and Weber, M. (2017), "My Health Record: The resuscitation of e-health, or a data placebo?", Image & Data Manager, 13 April 2017, Online Available at:

https://idm.net.au/article/0011469-my-health-record-resuscitation-e-health-or-data-placebo (accessed on 10 May 2017).

Thompson, R. L., Higgins, C. A. and Howell, J. M. (1991), "Personal computing: toward a conceptual model of utilization", MIS Quarterly, Vol. 15, No. 1, pp. 125-143.

Thurston, J. (2014), "Meaningful use of Electronic Health Records", The Journal of Nursing Practitioners, Vol. 10, Issue 7, pp. 510-513.

Venkatesh, V. and Davis, F. D. (2000), "A theoretical extension of the technology acceptance model: four longitudinal field studies", Management Science, Vol. 46, No. 2, pp. 186-204.

Xu, J. and Quaddus, M. (2007), "Exploring the Factors Influencing End Users' Acceptance of Knowledge Management Systems: Development of a Research Model of Adoption and Continued Use", Journal of Organizational and End-Users Computing, Vol. 19, No.4, pp. 57-79.

Xu. J. and Quaddus, M. (2009) ed., E-Business in the 21st Century: Realities, Challenges, and Outlook, World Scientific, Singapore.

Xu, J., Gao, X., and Sorwar, G. (2014), "A research model of consumers' adoption and continued use of the Personally Controlled Electronic Health Record (PCEHR) system", International Technology Management Review, Vol. 4, No.4, pp. 187-200.

Xu, J., Gao, X., Sorwar, G. and Croll, P. (2012), "Current Status, Challenges, and Outlook of E-Health Record Systems in Australia", 7th International Conference on Intelligence Systems and Knowledge Engineering, Dec 15-17, 2012, Beijing, China.

Xu, J., Gao, X., Sorwar, G. and Croll, P. (2013), "Implementation of E-Health Record Systems in Australia", International Technology Management Review, Vol. 3, No.2, pp. 92-104.

Zmud, R. W. (1979), "Individual differences and MIS success: a review of the empirical literature", Management Science, Vol. 25, No. 10, pp. 966-979.

Chapter 2

Field Studies of Personal Electronic Health Record System Users in Australia

This chapter looks at the understanding of and the current status of adoption and use of the personally controlled electronic health record (PCEHR) system among Australian consumers and Australian doctors and aims to identify concerns/issues associated with the PCEHR system and factors influencing their decision regarding adoption and use of the PCEHR system. Qualitative field studies were undertaken, in which 30 consumers/individual users and 10 doctors were interviewed.

Keywords: PCEHR System, My Health Record, Adoption & Use, Consumers, Doctors, Australia, Field Studies

2.1 Introduction

The current release of the PCEHR system in Australia is far from mature and suffers criticisms from major stakeholders, and there is a lack of uptake and utilization (Partel 2015). The system is facing various challenges, and users are not enthusiastic in registering with and using the system (Sansom 2016; Swinn & Weber 2017). Participation in the PCEHR system is essential for adoption and use of the system. Consumers have not been active in participation for different reasons and various concerns. The interests of consumers have been properly represented in the development and implementation of the PCEHR system. In the PCEHR review ordered by the Coalition Government in 2013, no review panel members are really representing consumers. Moreover, there is a lack of comprehensive empirical studies on the current status, challenges/issues, as well as success factors and failure reasons of the PCEHR system uptake and use by the individual users (i.e., consumers).

Even though the Australian government has invested significantly in deploying the system and its associated infrastructure (including required technological infrastructure, standards, legislations, and others), but the system has not been well received by users (including both consumers/individual users and health care providers). In addition, there is a lack of the comprehensive empirical studies of the current status and challenges/issues as well as the reasons and factors for success and failure of electronic health record systems, especially PCEHR (My Health Record). The study reported in this chapter fills the gap by studying the factors influencing the adoption and use of the PCEHR system by individual users/consumers and health care providers.

Data were collected by means of semi-structured interview. 30 selected eligible consumers (i.e., must be Australian Citizen or Permanent Resident) and 10 doctors were interviewed in Gold Coast and Brisbane areas. The interview plan followed the guidelines of Whiteley et al. (1998) and Patton (1990). The high-level perspective of external factors and internal factors in the model for adoption and use of the PCEHR system by Xu et al. (2014) discussed in Chapter 1 guided the entire interview process. Interview questions were first developed and tested by third parties. The interview questions focused on: (i) the general perceptions and understanding of the PCEHR system; (ii) the current status of adoption and use of the system; (iii) concerns and issues associated with system; (iv) obstacles to adopting the system; and (v) motivating factors for adopting and use the system.

A pre-interview session was first conducted through telephone, which provided each participant with an idea about the interview process. Content analysis (Berg 2001) was chosen for analyzing the interview transcripts. Content analyses were carried out in two stages (Miles & Huberman 1994). Stage one dealt with single interview transcripts and developed tables of factors, variables and their links for each interview; and stage two focused on analysing cross-interview transcripts and worked on integrating all the individual factors, variables and their relationships to come up with a final list of factors and variables as well as their links.

2.2 Results

2.2.1 Demographic Information

Of the 30 consumer interview participants, 16 are females and 14 are males. 3 participants are in the 21-29 age group, 8 in the age group of 30-39, 5 in the age group of 40-49, 4 in age group of 50-59, 5 in the age group of 60-64, and 5 over 65. Two participants are Aboriginal Australian or Torres Strait Islander. 24 participants have at least a Bachelor's degree, with 13 having Bachelor's Degree, 5 having Graduate Certificate or Graduate Diploma, 5 having a Master's degree, and 1 having a Doctorate's degree. The distribution of the participants by occupation/profession is as follows: 5 retired, 2 IT professionals, 2 nurses, 1 pharmacist, 1 teacher, 1 self-employed, 1 mortician, 1 student, 1 marketing professional, 1 consultant, 1 home duties, 1 travel agent, 1 public servant, 1 fulltime carer, 1 bus driver, 1 executive legal secretary, 1 trainer and assessor, 1 HRM professional, 1 accountant, 1 draftsperson, 1 office manager/secretary, 1 carpenter, 1 unemployed, and 1 transport industry employee. 3 Participants have registered with PCEHR system, 3 have e-health experience, and 25 have experience with other government systems (e.g., Census and MyGov). Meanwhile only 3 participants have obtained information about the PCEHR system (i.e., having seen/read writing in the newspaper, having seen advertising in the doctor's office, and/or having been provided with brochures by the doctor's receptionist).

Of the 10 doctor interview participants, 5 are female and 5 are male. 2 participants are in the 21-29 age group, 1 in the age group of 30-39, 4 in the age group of 40-49, 1 in age group of 50-59, and 2 in the age group of 60-69. 4 have less than 5-years GP experience, 2 with 5-10 years, 1 with 15-20 years, and 3 with more than 20 years. 3 have their own practice.

2.2.2 Consumers' Understanding of PCEHR System

Consumers participating the interview reported various understanding of PCEHR System (see Table-1).

Table-1: Australian Consumers' Understanding of PCEHR System

- "It is an electronic register to record kept medical details about self as transportable platform if you change GP.
- It is an electronic health record for health profession to maintain a record for other health professionals to access and update with 24/7 access and availability.
- It is an electronic record of my health records.
- Everyone has national record that can be accessed. Centralised health records.
- A record of people's health history in one place.
- It is a way of having all the medical people you see record your information in one place.
- All doctors having access to all medical history.
- I have some sort of control over what is in the system and who gets it and who sees it.
- Government run database which has information about health. Kept apart from others and some people have access to see my medical data.
- Doctors computerising health information and collated into a database regarding the health of the nation.
- Central database of personal records accessed by someone else.
- I know it exists. For different medical centres to share my medical records.
- System that keeps a record of medical history irrespective of who the provider was.

• A system that holds everything like vaccinations, medical records as my health history. The system permits doctors to see the history. • The collection of medical records of a person by a government body. Records such as blood tests, scans, operations and the reports/results interpreted by cardiologists, specialist, and GP. They can be accessed by all qualified parties that are involved in the wellbeing of that person readily available electronically. • When attending doctors, they can upload your history record to something like MyGov wherein your details can be accessed by other permitted professionals (or potentially hackers) and maybe yourself. • I have heard about PCEHR through doctors at the Wesley Hospital in the last 12 months. I believe it to be a collection of data referring to my medical history that can be accessed nationally. • Keeping health records nationwide and having access to it (doctors and allied professionals only)."

(Source: Developed for this study)

2.2.3 Views on PCEHR System Characteristics/Features

Table-2 presents individual consumers' views on PCEHR system characteristics/features/factors while Table-3 shows doctors' perspectives of PCEHR system characteristics/features/factors.

Table-2: Consumers' Views

Views/Perspectives	Quotations from Interview Participants
Option to test the system before registration	• "Any good system should be fully tested, e.g., testing privacy and security so why use dummy data to learn the system. • Just to see how it works. • That would be great."
Linking PCEHR system worldwide	• "Just Australia. Could have opt-in as part of travel/health insurance. • Absolutely. Also travel insurance need to access/view to determine pre-existing conditions. • No. What happens in Australia stays in Australia. • Yes for a hospital only. • It would be a useful benefit or desirable. • Yes as long as privacy is addressed. • No. Should not have automatic access but can request it. • No but possibly with some protocols in place. • Yes if guarantee of security and privacy. Just treatment data should be transmitted to Australia in pdf format.

	• Yes because it would make it easier but NO because you need protocols. • Yes provided they have authority. • Yes - travel benefits. • Yes. It would be very useful if I was ever overseas."
Public sector working with Private sector for the greater good of the system	• "I would like to think so. Not sure about efficiencies, there is room for improvement. • Theoretically great but unlikely. • Depends on the cost. If private sector paid to use system, then they should work together. • All control and access so they probably need to work together. • Hope so but not sure. • No but they should. • They can but believe not 100%. • They could if they wanted to. • Doubt it unless a lot of money is given to both."
Users' Attitude towards PCEHR System and the Government	• "Users' doctor (GP) has significant influence on their adoption (registration) decision of the PCEHR system: "I am going to register next time I visit the GP. If he is not of the opinion to register, then ask him for reasons and then make a decision." • Don't trust government: "Very sceptical about Government control over my personal medical data." • Lack of information and knowledge of the system: "Why are there not brochures available for people"; "It would have been nice to have some information about the system….." • Security concerns: "Only other concerns are cyber-attacks, potential threats of hacking. So, need to address this. The census was a disaster." • Privacy issues: "I would love my information in one database but worry about privacy." • Involvement of insurance firms: "Insurance company needs to be involved where overseas medical problem arises and (it) needs to check previously existing condition."
Rules for managing data change in the system	• "There should be protocols for any change for everyone who can access. • Approval by third party or the GP for all changes made by all who access.

	• There should be strict guidelines in place for complete privacy. • Rules should be approved by Board of Practitioners. • I should make the rules. • When changes are made I should be notified. • All changes should be approved by a second party OR reviewed by third party. All changes should be approved by patient. Changes by YOU (need to be) approved by GP. • Changes should be approved by patient and GP or head nurse or third party. • All changes reviewed by third parties. • For changes by hospital, than approved by GP. For changes by allied health, then approved by GP. • Changed by GP for basic changes are OK. If major changes then depends what the major change is. Same for hospital. Changes by YOU - No, but there should be a right to query information. • GP and other medical related people, then just change. Changes by YOU to be approved by GP. • If GP, then no rules. If by hospital or nurses, then approved by case manager. If by others e.g. physio, then no authority to change. By YOU - not acceptable. • If by GP, don't know if we need rules. If by hospital, approved by patient. If by YOU - no change - restricted changes. • If by GP - not sure. If changed by hospital then GP. If changed by others then GP. If changed by YOU - no changes. • If changed by GP or hospital then no rules for authority. GP has over-riding authority. If changed by YOU - approved by GP in comments or feedback. • If change by GP, the approval by patient. Same for hospital and other medical. If changed by YOU, approval by GP or hospital. • For changes by GP and specialists, then no rules needed. (Changed by)YOU - need approval by GP. • For changes to be made, the reason should be recorded and by whom. Only GP should change data. YOU - only change address, phone numbers and that's all. • If changes by GP or hospital, then need to notify the patient and all other parties. If changed by YOU, then need approval by other parties. Data needs to be consistent.

	• General staff able to change on advice of medical professionals. Changes by YOU should only limit to personal contact details".

(Source: Developed for this study)

Table-3: Doctors' Views

Views/Perspectives	Quotations from Interview Participants
Clarification of information required for the system	"The system is good. But I think we need to know what sort of information we need to upload. What important information we need to upload. Let's say we can upload the last blood tests in the last year, the last blood tests for the patient, last screening or testing like bowel cancer screen test, mammogram, pap smears. This important information is last ones which any doctor can build from this last one onwards. That's important."
Completeness of the Information in the System	"They do say that the blood results and radiology and everything else will be eventually included. I'm not sure if that is already in the system. So those are the ones that would definitely help us, especially if there is any hospital x-ray or CT scans that are done. Sometimes we don't get it in the discharge summaries so if that is accessible. Blood tests again, we don't really get in the discharge summary. If those are accessible to us, it will help and also medications. That's another thing. Pharmacies. If they are involved in the system. If there is a system we can actually get which pharmacy the patient has gone and have a list as to what medication especially the codeine drugs, opioids, being included would help us a lot. And see how many times the patient has gone to get medications and their antibiotic pills etc. So I think that is important."
Currency of the information in the system.	"…concerns about it actually being updated in a timely fashion."
Having a mobile application for the system	"Having an iPhone app would be awesome for everyone. So if you have a My Health Record, having an app for easier access. …The iPhone accessibility for patients might improve the ability of patients to keep their medical records up to date and also help for older folks. An iPhone is more intuitive that a desk top system so therefore better for people to keep their records up to date."
Linking to state government's health systems	"As a doctor, I can get most of the information from Qld Health which I prefer. We access hospital discharge reports via a QLD Health portal. It is not everyone accessing it. I need to be told by a patient that they attended hospital and then I access the portal to read and download the report. The report is not sent automatically to the patient's doctor. This is preferred."
Digitizing the doctor's summary notes	"…ask the doctor if he was more conscious about what he writes in his notes. He stated that they are just summaries and not very detailed. He has always done this and will continue. So the eHealth has not changed what he writes."
Simplicity	"Sometimes when we ring to get information from another doctor, another GP, whatever like this. They don't like it if they ....too

	many steps, too many questions. It is unrealistic, taking time so we got a lot of patients to care about. It needs to very smooth, very simple, streamlined."
Organization of the information in the system	"At the moment, there are not much help from usually … I would like to see the clear diagnosis on their regular medication but it was not the case. Sometimes there are too many complicated hospital reports are not much help"
Compatibility	"I think the biggest one would be, like me having to go to an external source, like go online, login and that sort of stuff. It's not compatible with the software that I have. …No there is not."
Special treatment & Protection for certain personal information	"…So patients being able to see it, I would even omit certain things because it would be not well received. Yeah. I would be a little cautious about recording sexual and drug history and stuff like that".
Speed	"Yes. As I said, it's the speed. Usually it's getting populated very quickly so you do see prescriptions pop up reasonably quickly. So the lab results are starting to come and be more useful. Still seeing a lot of patchiness. …I have to say that they [tests] seem to be much slower than prescriptions which I think the pharmacists are probably already on to it as its going to help them. So they're in to it. I think one of the biggest problems is just the specialists. They just have not got around to it. They are often running the important tests. I don't care about their letters."
Exclusion of certain sensitive personal information	"No. I have to say … they don't work unless they are opt out. The same as cervical screening. There are other ones for years we tried opt in, and I suppose it's like donors…"
Interoperability	"…I think and I know that there are programs supposedly out there where interoperability is really important and trying to get platforms that can translate information from one system into another into its fields. So you don't get loss of data or it's gone to the wrong place, you can't find it, or those sorts of things.…They are so full of added on bits and pieces and that's just really annoying. There are certain things that could have been fixed and could have been made more interoperable…And we know there are such amazing systems out there. Why they're not actually. I think they need a hand from the government systems, all of these things, Centrelink, the whole lot, needs to be much more modernized."
Ease of Use/User friendliness	"I'm not an IT specialist, but I found the system friendly to use. It's easy to use and hopefully our clients will continue using it."

(Source: Developed from Xu et al. 2021)

2.2.4. Expected Benefits

Table-4 presents individual consumers' perceived/expected benefits of the PCEHR system while Table-5 shows doctors' perspectives of perceived/expected benefits of the PCEHR system.

Table-4 Consumers' Views

Views/Perspectives	Quotations from Interview Participants
Better medical/health information	"Know that records kept electronically secure. Accurate data"; "Permanent record of health of the nation"; "Greater access in

management:	remote areas. Information all in the one place and current"; "Benefit where you forget medical history"; "Continuity of record keeping. Moving house / divorce. Forget data especially trying to remember data for children"; "Information shared so that you don't have to go through your entire medical history each time"; "Have data that can look afresh at problem i.e. complete picture"; "Comprehensive record of medical history of the family"; "GP have better picture of my overall health. Good when I change GPs or go to specialists and not have to explain everything. Knowing when my last episode or flare up was, so I can be informed as with all my medications I get foggy on dates, etc."
Faster and better access to the medical/health information	"One central body holding all the information. All relevant health issues available to the GP. Distance is no problem especially for the traveller. Speed of access of information if records are categorized properly"; "Being able to access any time if needed. Being able to view updates from other parties. Used for follow-up of conditions"; "Access to the data nationally. Don't have to repeat yourself and medical history at every visit. Good for contact details in an emergency".
Better healthcare services and system	"Improve patient care and speed"; "Greater health outcomes "Better health care. With NBN, larger data e.g. X-rays can be sent quickly. Safer if all records are up to date"; "Overall the system should become more efficient for everyone"; "Better services"; "Holistic approach to healthcare. Treating professionals have complete health record. More efficient diagnosis and less bed time which leads to critical diagnosis and targeted treatments quicker"; "Good for ambulance and emergency services having immediate access to your information"; "Provide more accurate diagnosis or problem therefore quicker diagnosis and quicker treatment, quicker recovery, and quicker return to work".
More streamlined processes	"Stop doctor shopping. No getting drugs from more than one doctor"; "Stops the need for letters and referrals"; "Ease in transferring GPs".
Better health awareness	"More awareness of your health. Get alerts"; "Stop multiple visits and have an audit trail of visits".
Cost reduction and time saving	"Reduced costs. Getting medical history faster"; "Should save time and doctor should run on time as all information presented".
Economic benefits	"Economic benefit leading to lower cost of delivery leading to cost efficiencies".
Mobility	"Mobility. Able to look up dates (of conditions) as system accessible".
Research and Trend Identification and Disease Prevention	"Ability to develop trends. Big data to highlight ailments by age or postcode. Record of health medications prescribed"; "Research more into certain things like vaccinations"; "Big data analysis"; "Government and research industry with medical records available as a tool for research"; "Definitely research and more information on what is being done in my illness. Being informed is very important to me"; "Disease prevention and tracking".
Mistake Reduction	"Help save mistakes e.g. wrong drugs given".
Better Communication	"Communication between all healthcare providers. Deliver health

between Healthcare Providers	benefits leads to economic benefits to the Australian community".

(Source: Developed for this study)

Table-5 Doctors' Views

Views/Perspectives	Quotations from Interview Participants
Accessing patient medical/health information anytime anywhere	"If they don't have an eHealth record, we always suggest to them to have an eHealth record because they may be travelling all over Australia and easy for any doctor to have a look after their approval."
Accessing new patient information faster with better efficiency	"We see new patients every day and these new patients have health records which we don't know anything about them. And the health records are normally in the old practices or in other practices. So in order to know their information, we have to send a consent (paper or fax) to other clinic and wait for about 2 to 4 weeks and have another reply. If the patient has an eHealth record, it just takes about 10 minutes to check what he's having, what sort of medication, what sort of problems, to give us a better idea how we can manage the patient on past history and present complaint."
Providing more accurate and complete information than the patient can provide.	"Easier access especially any medication change, any blood results, etc. Because patients do not remember their medications easily and overall safer practice."
Speed (in terms of uploading & getting the required information.	"Yes. As I said, it's the speed. Usually it's getting populated very quickly so you do see prescriptions pop up reasonably quickly."
Without reinventing the wheel & avoiding doubling up	"…There are certain tests you would have to re-order anyway. But sometimes, yes, we are ordering the same things because we don't have a record and we need to know it. So it would probably save money, not every time but it would in some instances"
Providing a broad and more complete picture about the patient & thus achieving proper diagnosis & medication and treatment plan	"It saves time, gives us a broad picture about the patient, past history, medical conditions, medications, help us to reach proper diagnosis, know more about him, and their health."
Reducing conflicts & having better way to manage the patient.	"Saves lots of conflicts (from different sources) we can have. Phone calls speaking to nurses, other nurses, other clinics, other pharmacies….It will give us a better way to manage the patient."
Making decision better and easier	"If you have proper information, you make a diagnosis decision. If lack of information, you can't do anything. But you need time to make that decision. If you have that information available to you, it will help you to make decision better and easier."
Providing better explained and more updated information by both the doctor and the patient.	"Clarity of information from both sides. Doctors obviously then will be forced to update their summaries regularly"
Keeping the patient's medical/health information	"It basically is making us clean out everybody's past medical, unwanted past medical history, unwanted medications, etc.

accurate, organized and updated via cleaning out unwanted information.	So from time to time, that is a benefit to clean up a person's record and make sure everything is up to date."
Having easier access to the required information	"It really depends you know. It's helpful if they go from one doctor to other doctor or go to the hospital. It's easier access to the information rather than the hospital calling us to find the information about the patient".
Improving the quality of the patient's care as a system approach	"I see the system of primary benefit for the patients themselves. And so the intention is to improve the quality of their care as a systems approach and not just here. The flow through effects I haven't seen a whole lot of benefits just yet in terms of me accessing information I wouldn't have had access to otherwise for patients who are interstate, etc."
Being ideal for patients traveling interstate for an extended period of time	"No. Not really, very rarely and that's if they are travelling interstate for an extended period of time."
Enabling continuity of care (especially for those patients who see multiple doctors)	"Continuity of care especially for those patients who see multiple doctors."
Benefiting some patients with critical medical conditions more than others	"I use it for some patients, those with critical medical conditions who might (be frequent visitors) of hospitals. It is more important to these patients for their medical care."
Accessing the information in an emergency situation	"I think it is important to have medical information available in an emergency where the patient cannot talk and answer questions. So for those elderly patients who might have a fall and go to hospital, then it is important that they get the best care."
Reducing the admin workload	"I guess it's similar to practitioners like the practice gets more updated medical information and I guess from like the other admin work side it might reduce their workload. They don't have to go around chasing things, like bloods, if we already have it on the eHealth system."

(Source: Developed from Xu et al. 2021)

2.2.5. Concerns & Issues

Table-6 provides consumers' concerns & issues of the PCEHR system while Table-7 presents doctors' concerns & issues of the PCEHR system.

Table-6 Consumers' Views

Views/Perspectives	Quotations from Interview Participants
The Impact of Continuity of the Government	• "The change in the government could result in the cut in spending and staffing of the system. • New government may want to change things. • Change of mind comes with the change of the government."
Reasons for not registering with the PCEHR system	• "Lack of information and knowledge about the system: "Not seen any information and therefore not registered. Did not know about the system"; "Government fraud. Not trust government. Information may end up in the wrong hands";

	"Not know much about it. Need more information before making a decision"; "Don't read material in mail that was not addressed to me. (If not addressed to me, I think of it as junk mail and throw it out.). Hate reading screens of information": "The great unknown - know nothing about the system"; "No knowledge about it". • Lack of awareness. • Apathy/Lack of interest. • Lack of required computer skills. • Aversion to computer systems or Don't trust computers. • Lack of established access protocols. • Time poor or being lazy: "No time"; "Too lazy - not enough time and effort". • Lack of opportunity: "Not really have any medical issues"; "Don't go the GP often". • Lack of necessity: "My GP already has enough information regarding my health". • General ignorance of the users by the government. • Privacy concerns and security of system: "Seen many cases when information leaked. Concerns over who can access. Concerns over ability to save data". • No Trust towards the government: "Sceptical. No confidence in the Government to pull this off. If they cannot run the country successfully, then how can they pull this off?"; "Government fraud. Not trust government. Information may end up in the wrong hands".
Concerns over the ability to access and save information in the system	• "Major concern as to the saving of data to mobile devices. • Should be viewable but not downloadable. • Should not be able to save to personal devices. • Not to saving the data. If this is needed, then get permission based on reason. • No concerns to view/download. It should not be saved. • Should have read only access and should have no ability to save. • Can save data for treatments is OK; for general research then No. Have concerns that Insurance firms could access without individual's knowledge. • No concerns except download to personal devices. Must be to non-personal devices. • Concerns over privacy and security. • Some concerns over potential hackers but this is a small threat.

	• I wouldn't want my private health information seen by others other than health practitioners."
Trusting GP and other healthcare providers to update information	• "Yes trust the GP but not trust the Government system • GPs already complain about doing unfunded work. They want to be reimbursed for this duty. • Yes but only important information required (to be put into the system)."

(Source: Developed for this study)

Table-7 Doctors' Views

Views/Perspectives	Quotations from Interview Participants
Patient's consent/Approval	"We're speaking about confidentiality. What the patients want to do. So if the patient wants their medical records to be on the system. But if the patient does not want it, then we have to state that."
Being hesitant to put all the information into the system as a result of privacy concerns	"…Not for me, but for some patients – they do concern about the privacy, privacy issues of their information. They could be sometime hesitant to put all their information onto the system."
The impacts of security concerns on young families	"Security of the system is probably the main one. And most of my patients - I have a high proportion of young families and they are twice as hesitant to use the My Health Record just because of the security issues."
Control of access to the system	"So the things I have already mentioned - so the safety, the lack of control of who uses or accesses that information…."
Due diligence in terms of consent	"I think it should have been an opt-in system because the government does not have informed consent from people about the collection and the storing of their sensitive personal medical information. And they can't tell me that they have done due diligence in terms of consent."
Third parties (such as insurance companies) accessing the information in the system	"There is talk about insurance companies having access or wanting access to the records for insurance purposes. Not too sure about this."
Concerns of Extra consideration of confidentiality	"…One is patient confidentiality. It is an unnecessary extra consideration. So we do need to trust each other in health provision. There is no need to be … extra consideration of confidentiality."
Privacy Education by Privacy Commission	"…They need to address the privacy, The Privacy Commission, they can educate a lot."
Safeguarding healthcare service providers from potential unnecessary legal implications arising from privacy issues	"We as health care providers need a safeguard doing it in good faith, for the best benefit of the patient."
Providing no personal comments on patient medical conditions & health	"Yes. I think both (threat of being sued and being cautious). Like if another health practitioner has used my notes, there is always that concern that judgment and whatever, what I've

information	written is medically sound, and even from the patient's point of view, sometimes I will write patient's specific comments maybe about their behaviour which, you have to be careful cause if the patient can read it, they may get upset. So always having to word things so it's not sounding personal."
Young patients' concerns of access to their sensitive medial information by their parents	" ...I certainly do have patients where I've got 2 very antagonistic parents and their children's notes were a possible way for them finding out about the other parent and also young women who need contraception or perhaps even abortion services who's biggest problem is about relatives knowing. I am very keen they can't be accessed once it's becoming clearer that young women ... their parents could not get into their notes and definitely no confidentiality breach, then I was much happier to encourage people to get on the system."

(Source: Developed from Xu et al. 2021)

2.2.6 System Use and Success

Table-8 lists consumers' views of system use & success of the PCEHR system while Table-9 spells out doctors' views of system use & success of the PCEHR system.

Table-8 Consumers' Views

Views/Perspectives	Quotations from Interview Participants
Reasons for support of the influence of their age on the adoption and use of the system	• "If younger, then younger people don't seem to care about Govt. As you get older, you get more health problems. Also as you get older, you become aware of government problems. • The older you get, you get more medical problems. • Yes due to my aversion to computers. • Yes as I don't use computers that much. • Absolutely. I am not electronically minded. • The older you get, the more likely to seek medical assistance. Enormous help as you get older to remember history of overall health (i.e., Preventative rather than immediate treatment). • More inclined to use it as in IT and if I had medical issues. • At my age I loathe the computer with passwords more and more. • Younger people more likely to use the system - more accepting."
Reasons for supporting compulsory registration	• "Wider benefit for society. Reduced cost. Consistent access to data for all Australians. • Otherwise why have an incomplete system. • Holistic approach needs to be registered. Cost efficient.

	• It will be easier and more functional if all in the system. • What is the point of the system if not everyone is in the system. • More meaningful for overall public benefit. Lower cost. Better healthy lifestyle. • Makes it easier for doctors to run on time if they have all your history. Doctors can find the information easier and therefore quicker treatment. • More beneficial is all are registered. • Handy to have everyone registered. • Health concerns are a public problem. Someone has a right to know if they are treating a person with a contagious or life-threatening ailment. • If the system is proven to work, and easy to use, then for Aussie's overall health. • Easy when moving GP."
Reasons given by participants for against compulsory registration	• "The system is broken/incomplete - too many problems at present. Rules need to be finalised. • Should have choice to register or not; People should have a choice. • It is an individual decision; Up to each individual - personal choice; Should be an individual choice just like health insurance; Individual has rights as to what they want to do with their own information. • People still need freedom to deal with data in their own way. • Don't like compulsory requirements; Not a fan of compulsory conditions / more optional. • Personal reason not to be in the system, e.g., distrust of government (i.e., Big brother). • Like to see it compulsory but there should be free choice. • There is a lot of personal information that may be sensitive".

(Source: Developed for this study)

Table-9 Doctors' Views

Views/Perspectives	Quotations from Interview Participants
Quick and proper implementation	"From my experience here in general practice, any new applications need to be applied quickly and in a proper way…"
Nothing stopping the users to use the system	"I don't see that. I don't think there should be any problems here as such. I can't see any problems like technology or anything like that

	t is going to stop us from using the system here in this clinic."
Helping both patients and doctors	"Same, exactly the same reasons. (We will continually use the system). It just helps both patients and doctors dealing with actual patient."
Positive user feedback	"It all depends on how the system goes. I haven't heard any bad, any negative feedback from the patients yet. It all depends."
No complaints for the system.	"I don't see any at the moment. Because we are still in the initial stages and we can see the benefits of the system. I don't think we have a lot of complaints about that. Mostly people are happy with the system when we talk to them. These are the benefits so they are happy with the system. There might be some people concerned about it but I haven't, I didn't come across yet any particular concerns from the patients."
Keeping on using the system as long as it can deliver benefits.	"That depends on the system which continues to change. But if it continues to remain a benefit, then I expect so."
Network effects	"Having enough patients who are enrolled in the system and are actually using it, means you are more likely to use it often and be familiar with it and navigate your way around it. But one patient in a million using it probably won't be proficient at using it."
Critical mass	"The system is only good if the majority of patients are in the system. If very few are in the system, then it is a bit worthless."
Patients' needs & care	"We are starting to become ... we are expecting to just … especially with the patients, they say can you just look at my notes and see if my records got it in. So that's enough incentive for us to keep going because patients are going to expect it. We have led them to expect that as well."

(Source: Developed from Xu et al. 2021)

2.2.7 Doctor and Clinic Factors

Factors related to doctor and clinic are reported in Table-10.

Table-10 Doctor and Clinic Factors

Views/Perspectives	Quotations from Interview Participants
Doctor's failing to learn the system	"…(One of the barriers is) Just failing to learn the system"
Doctor's negative attitude towards eHealth system	"Doctors don't want the eHealth system and the doctors are the rubber on the road."
Doctor's computing skill	"On a practice level, if some of the doctors are not that familiar with using computers, or getting the access, then that would prevent other doctors."
Practice/Clinic's RCGP (Royal College of General Practitioners) Accreditation requirements	"I know it is one of the requirements for accreditation of the RSGP or clinic and practices to encourage doctors to upload the eHealth records of the patients."
Uncertainty in relations with the federal government	"I am OK with the Queensland Health having access to medical records. We have got a high degree of being able to influence a local state government. Our ability to influence the doings or the not doings or federal government is less. I don't want to give sensitive information or have my patients give sensitive to a

	government which we don't have as much control over as we would like."
Having no confidence/trust towards the federal government (like a revolving government)	"Yes. With the government, there is knee-jerk reaction. They change things all the time. It seems to change with the wind and that's a lot of control to give to a federal government that you don't have that much control over."
Variances in the federal government	"…and the variances (frequent changes) of the federal government (discourage the adoption/use of the system)."
Negative news on media	"What I don't like about the system. I think just the recent news about My Health Records and things like that and to make sure the safety of it not being leaked. To a third party. I think they are the things that are discouraging rather than anything else like negative news that comes on the radio is not going to help us help patients."
Peer influence	"I suppose it's a bit of peer influence as the surgery wants to be more efficient, not spend time looking up results and trying to get results and information from hospitals and previous GPs. So there is that."
Demand from patients	"….I think it's a bit harder for older people and that's where they need a practice to access it for them and help them…"
Practice's support (technological infrastructure) to the system	"Yeah look I think. I can only speak for myself but also in general, GPs are often quite busy and there are only so many things you can provide your attention to. Some things that helped bring my attention to using the electronic health record has been, being aware of how to access it through our particular software platform in this practice and I know there have been broader incentives to register people for the electronic health record. That's something I am aware of through our practice."
Organizational initiatives of promoting & monitoring the adoption of the system	"We have tried to keep, initially, a tally of how we are going with, having people registered for the electronic health record as a way of improving self-awareness of whether or not we are having that discussion with patients. So they're probably things that bring it to my attention and made it easier to use or become familiar with the system."
Organizational efforts of developing awareness of the system.	"Probably has something to do with the awareness that I have about it in general as part of the practice policies sort of thing."
Monitoring the adoption and usage of the system	"…as I have said, we do keep, or initially we were keeping a tally as we do in terms of other, not so much audits, but we like to keep a check every now and then of how we are doing, for want of a better term, KPIs, and that was one thing we focused on over a period of time as to how we were tracking utilizing electronic health records. It just makes you more aware of it when we bring it up in discussion."
Organization's approach of asking chronic disease patients to adopt the system	"We do try and ask them (chronic disease patients) through general practice management plan time because they are the ones with the chronic illnesses so the nurses will often get the notes and get them all ready."
Organization's culture and support to the system	"Anecdotally, I don't know. From the beginning of the year, where it was just blanked out. There's just about always

	something in the slot now so I think that is due to the practice manager being ready and the staff making sure that everyone's asked about it. And it's either red, they have definitely opted out already or it's green and there is some information there. So I think we are doing pretty well."

(Source: Developed from Xu et al. 2021)

2.2.8 Facilitating and Support Factors

Facilitating and support factors to the implementation of the PCEHR system are reported in Table-11.

Table-11 Facilitating and Support Factors

Views/Perspectives	Quotations from Interview Participants
Compensation for the time spending on uploading the information into the system	"The only issue is billing for this consultation. Because Medicare does not bill us or pay for us to do this consultation. Normally we have a separate consultation for the patient and we have to upload the information in which he agrees for us to upload. It is not a clinical problem. It is just uploading information, technically, so the Medicare does not pay for that for us. So we are struggling about Medicare."
More publicity, communication and education of the system	"The only barriers is that I think that you need more publicity, more conversations, more conversations with the patients, more conversations on media, what benefits."
Incentive to use the system	"Yes. Of course. If there is an incentive then sure I'll go for it."
Patient's health and care being more important than incentive	"I don't really bother about that (the incentive program like ePIP). I don't really look at that. I just talk to the patient and in regards to their health and how important it is to get it across to other teams of the medical profession rather than how much money or what incentive there is."
Sufficient training	"It's not that we…. It's just that we didn't have enough training on time to use it today as such."
Time to learn and use the system	"I would like to put more on the system but it takes time to learn and upload."
Promotion, assistance and encouragement by the practice	"Oh yeah. Definitely. If you go out in the waiting room and have a look, there are some posters. Posters for the patients how to enrol onto the system and what are the benefits and if they have any difficulty, where they can seek help. They can ask the nursing staff. They can ask the doctors. We have all got quite reasonable information about how to enrol the patient to the system, how to use and what are the benefits. Yes, and all the nurses, when they see the nurses, nursing staff as well. So again we try to get in in a limited amount of time to get the information to the patient. We have leaflets, pamphlets, and things. We give to patients to go home and read it, and come back

	with any questions."
Conflicts of interest imposed by financial incentives	"I guess in some ways you might call it a conflict of interests. The point of the incentives being there is to encourage practitioners to encourage patients to be part of the system which goes some way towards influencing people to make a decision perhaps above and beyond a decision they might have made based on their own understanding of the risks and benefits which in some sense is coercive. So from that sort of moralistic or ethical point of view perhaps it shouldn't be there but I understand that encouraging health practitioners to adopt changes is not an easy thing. Generally the idea of making health information accessible to people is a good one."
Addressing such issues as unclear understanding of the scope of the system and access management via more promotion & education and more discussion and communication between the patient and the doctor/provider.	"I think probably the thing that is unclear is the scope of what is included in the electronic health record which is really quite minimal at the moment, and my understanding of what is going to be included in the future… I'm a bit unaware of what is intended and how far it will go. Certainly in some of the discussion we hear about in the media, it sounds like there is a lot of anxiety about people accessing all of your health information and people seem unaware of the fact that for the health information to be there in the first place, someone has to upload a summary which is a decision made between the patient and their health care provider. And even when that summary is uploaded, it's a summary and not the contents of every consultation they have had. So that seems to be an area that doesn't seem to be well publicized and can be improved on, I guess."
Better incentive for uploading the information into the system	"It should definitely increase. We don't have time to upload...We need to be recompensed for the 5 to 10 minutes it takes us to do that."
Patient's computing skill	"But also you have patient factors. A lot of elderly patients who it would work for. But things like not having an iPhone, let alone the internet to connect to then to actually use the My Health system. This is the population that it is most likely to benefit yet they are the ones less likely to actually engage with it."
Awareness	"The biggest one is lack of awareness, it's something that is available for me to use as a GP. Probably the biggest one."
Assistance and training for doctors by the professional organization	"We haven't had any emails from any professional organisations about how to use it either".

(Source: Developed from Xu et al. 2021)

2.2.9 Doctor and Consumer/Patient Relation Factors

Factors related to doctor and patient/consumer relation is presented in Table-12.

Table-12 Doctor and Consumer/Patient Relation Factors

Views/Perspectives	Quotations from Interview Participants
Doctor's Recommendation to Patient	"If they don't have an eHealth record, we always suggest to them to have an eHealth record because they may be travelling all over Australia and easy for any doctor to have a look after their approval."
Doctor's Communication to Patient	"….we are speaking to patients about it, explaining the whole process, explaining about, explaining how it will help patients anywhere in Australia, and hoping outside of Australia one day…"
Doctor's support to stay in and not opt-out	"…I encourage always to be in. Because of their own benefits – health benefits. Situations like being travelling interstate, seeing doctors who doesn't know about him or her, about anything, how the medical records will help him to reach a proper diagnosis. It's very important."
Doctors' neutral stand	"I think for the patient, we should be neutral. Just tell them the advantages of opting in. And I don't think we should show any of our preferences to them and they should make the decision. And obviously give them the proper information and tell them what advantages are, and then they can make the decision."
Patients seeking guidance from their doctors	"As one of the GPs here, we are looking for patients coming to ask us to please upload my eHealth records and they sit with us and we discuss what information they want to be uploaded and what is the minimum information that should be uploaded. That would be good of course."
Doctor's support to opt-in approach	"I prefer opt-in to continue. It is a good system. They need to address the privacy…."
Doctor's support to opt-out approach	"What we have now is good because I think people who are highly motivated to opt-out because of the privacy concerns and information sharing and misuse, they are highly motivated so they're going to go to the effort to do that whereas your average person is not going to be motivated enough to opt-in whereas they might not actually care either way. So ultimately you would miss a lot of people if it was opt-in."

(Source: Developed from Xu et al. 2021)

2.3 Summary

This chapter reports results of field studies of consumers and doctors on their views of the implementation of personal electronic health record system (i.e., PCEHR system in Australia). Good understanding of users of the PCEHR system (including consumers and health care providers) could have significant contribution to the success of the PCEHR system in Australia.

Acknowledgement
This chapter is developed from the author's previous works: (1) "Understanding Individual

Users' Perspectives on the Personally Controlled Electronic Health Record (PCEHR) System: Results of Field Study", *Proceedings of 16th International Conference on Smart Homes, Assistive Technology and Health Telematics, Singapore*, 2018, pp.292-297; (2) "Doctors' Perspectives on Electronic Health Records: An Australian Study", in *E-Business in the 21st Century: Essential Topics & Studies*, pp. 143-168, World Scientific, Singapore.

References

Berg, B. L. 2001, Qualitative Research Methods for the Social Sciences, Allyn & Bacon, Boston.

Miles, M.B. & Huberman, M. A. 1994, An Expanded Sourcebook: Qualitative Data Analysis, 2nd Edition, SAGE Publications Thousands Oaks, California, USA.

Partel, K. 2015, "Toward better implementation: Australia's My Health Record", Deeble Institute Issues Brief, No. 13, 30/10/2015, pp.1-20.

Patton, Q.M. 1990, Qualitative Evaluation and Research Methods, 2nd Edition, Newbury Park: SAGE Publications.

Sansom, M. 2016, My Health Record: Medics speak up, Government News, 15 August 2016, Online Available at: http://www.governmentnews.com.au/2016/08/24703/ (accessed on 15 April 2017).

Swinn, M. & Weber, M. 2017, My Health Record: The resuscitation of e-health, or a data placebo?, Image & Data Manager, 13 April 2017, Online Available at: https://idm.net.au/article/0011469-my-health-record-resuscitation-e-health-or-data-placebo (accessed on 10 May 2017).

Xu, J., Gao, X., and Sorwar, G. 2014, "A research model of consumers' adoption and continued use of the Personally Controlled Electronic Health Record (PCEHR) system", International Technology Management Review , Vol.4, No.4, pp.187-200.

Xu, J., Gao, X., Sorwar, G., Hammond, J. & Antonius, N. 2021, "Doctors' Perspectives on Electronic Health Records: An Australian Study", in E-Business in the 21st Century: Essential Topics & Studies, eds. J. Xu, & X. Gao, pp. 143-168, World Scientific, Singapore.

Whiteley, A., McCabe, M., Buoy, L., Howie, F., Klass, D., Latham, J., Bickley, M. & Luckheenariam, L. 1998, Planning the Qualitative Research Interview, Working Paper Series 98.01, Graduate School of Business, Curtin University of Technology, Australia.

Chapter 3

Defining and Measuring Adoption and Continued Use of Personal Electronic Health Record System in Australia

This chapter discusses the development of the survey questionnaire of adoption and continued use of the PCEHR system in Australia, which includes sections of survey definitions, demographic information questions, questions on involvement in the PCEHR system, Questions on Current State of Adoption and Use of the PCEHR System, and Questions on Statements Regarding the PCEHR System. The questionnaire was developed based on the research model discussed in Chapter 1.

Keywords: PCEHR System, Adoption, Continued Use, Survey, Questionnaire, Australia.

3.1 Survey Definitions

The following definitions are adopted for the survey of Adoption and Continued Use of Personal Electronic Health Record System in Australia:

- ***Electronic Health (E-health):*** E-health is the electronic management of health information to deliver safer, more efficient, better quality healthcare.
- ***Electronic Health Records (EHRs):*** The electronic repositories of information regarding the health status of a subject of care, which can be managed electronically via Internet technologies and computing equipment.

- ***Electronic Medical Records (EMRs)***: In this study, electronic medical records are viewed as the equivalent of electronic health records, and they are used interchangeably.
- ***Personally Controlled Electronic Health Record (PCEHR)(Recently rebadged as "My Health Record") System***: A national wide personal electronic health record system rolled out on July 1, 2012 in Australia. The system can provide an online summary of an individual's health information. It is operated by the Department of Health, but an individual can control what goes into his/her health record and who is allowed to access it.
- ***Healthcare Providers:*** Including GPs, allied health professionals, medical specialists, pharmacies, hospitals (private and public), and other health/medical professions or institutions.
- ***Meaningful Use of the Information:*** Referring to what information is used by whom for what purpose on what occasion under what condition.

3.2 Demographic Information Questions

Questions for collecting respondents' demographic information are presented in Table-1, which include such perspectives as Gender, Age Group, Australian citizen or permanent resident of Australia, Aboriginal Australian or Torres Strait Islander, Post code in Australia, Highest level of education, Main profession or occupation, English language proficiency, Average weekly household income in the last financial year, Household composition, and Experience regarding E-health.

Table-1 Demographic Information Questions

Demographics	Survey Questions/Choices
Gender	• Male • Female
Age Group	• 18 - 20 • 21 to 29 • 30 to 39 • 40 to 49 • 50 to 59 • 60-65
Australian citizen or permanent resident of Australia	• Yes • No

Aboriginal Australian or Torres Strait Islander	• Yes • No
Post code in Australia	• Specify Post Code
Highest level of education	• Attended high school • Completed high school • Diploma • Bachelor's Degree • Graduate Certificate and Graduate Diploma • Master's Degree • Doctorate • Other (please specify)
Main profession or occupation	• Specify main profession or occupation
English language proficiency	• Native Speaker Able to communicate in both writing and speaking • Able to communicate in writing only • Able to communicate in speaking only • Other (please specify)
Average weekly household income in the last financial year	• Less than $401 $401 to 700 • $ 701 to 900 • $ 901 to 1,100 • $ 1,101 to 1,500 • $ 1,501 to 1,800 • More than $ 1,800
Household composition	• I am living in an aged care home (nursing home) • I am the only person • More than one person There is(are) newborn child(ren) • There is(are) child(ren) under the age of 14 • There is(are) a member(s) above 65 years old • There is(are) member(s) with chronic conditions, mental health conditions or disabilities • Other (please specify)
Experience regarding E-health	• I don't have any experience of E-health • I have experience of using telemedicine (i.e., enabling doctors and nurses to see and diagnose patients remotely) • I have experience of using electronic systems for healthcare supportive services (e.g., online appointment scheduling, checking in via kiosks, claiming expense online) • I have experience of participating in online health programs (e.g., health and fitness through diet and exercise programs)

	• I have experience of online treatments and assessments • I have experience of using health-related phone/tablets apps • I have experience of using wearable health and fitness tracking technology • Other (please specify)

3.3 Questions on Current State of Adoption and Use of the PCEHR System

Table-3 presents questions on current state of adoption and use of the PCEHR system, which look at such dimensions as: Have you registered for the PCEHR system? How long have you been registering for the system? How did you register for the PCEHR system? Where did you register for the PCEHR system? and What is your status of the actual use of the system?

Table-3 Current State of Adoption and Use Questions

Adoption and Use of the System	Survey Questions/Choices
Have you registered for the PCEHR system	• I will NOT register for the system • I don't know whether I will register for the system • I will register for the system • I have tried to register but experienced difficulties • I have registered for the system or on behalf of my dependant
How long have you been registering for the system	• Less than 1 month • More than 1 month but less than 3 months • More than 3 months but less than 6 months • More than 6 months but less than 12 months • More than 12 months but less than 18 months • More than 18 months but less than 24 months • More than 24 months but less than 36 months • I don't know • Other (please specify)
How did you register for the PCEHR system	• I registered myself • I registered with the assistance of the government departments or their agencies • I registered with the assistance of my GP • I registered with the assistance of other individuals (e.g., my friends, my family members) • Other (please specify)

Where did you register for the PCEHR system	• I registered • I registered over the phone • I registered via writing • I registered via Assisted Registration process • I registered at my GP's practice/clinic • I registered at the place of a healthcare provider (other than my GP) • I registered at a Medicare branch or other government agency office/branch • I registered at a mobile station/booth set up by the governments or their agencies • Other (please specify)
What is your status of the actual use of the system	• After registering with the system, I have not used the system at all • I don't know how to use the system • I have played around with the system, but have not really done anything yet • I have looked at and managed my records in the system along with my family • I have looked at and managed my records in the system along with my GP • I have looked at and managed my records in the system along healthcare providers (other than my GP) • I have used the system to some extent (e.g., uploading some information into the system) • I have used the system a lot and but still learning the system • I have used the system a lot and have known the system very well • Other (please specify)

3.4 Questions on Statements Regarding the PCEHR System

Table-4 indicates external factors & influences that could have impact on adoption and use of the PCEHR system. Respondents need to indicate the extent to which they agree with the following statements where 1 indicates that they strongly disagree with the statement and 7 indicates they strongly agree with the statement.

Table-4 Current State of Adoption and Use Questions

External Factors & Influences	Statements

Regulations and Policies	The regulations and policies relevant to the PCEHR system (e.g., Healthcare Identifiers Act 2010, Personally Controlled Electronic Health Records Act 2012) are essential to the implementation of the PCEHR system.
ICT Infrastructure Development	The deployment of national broadband and investments in e-heath infrastructure by federal and state governments have laid the foundation for the implementation of the PCEHR system.
Mobility	The increasing mobility of population from one place to another needs the PCEHR system so I can access my health information anywhere.
Availability of Computing Equipment and Popularity of Mobile Devices	The wide availability of computing equipment and the popularity of mobile devices have made the PCEHR system more popular.
Affordability and Accessibility of Internet Services	The high Internet penetration in Australia (more than 85%), as a result of good nationwide technology infrastructure and affordability, has made the PCEHR system more appealing.
Economic Uncertainty	The uncertainty of Australian economy will have impact on the future development of the PCEHR system.
Continuity of the Government	The instability of Federal and State governments will have an impact on the implementation of the PCEHR system.,
Unified Approach	Australia's multi-tier government system and large private sector has made the implementation of the PCEHR system extremely complex.
Transparency and Communication of The Operations of the PCEHR System	Improved transparency and communication regarding the operations of the PCEHR system could have positive impact on the implementation of the system.
Governance	Good governance model of the PCEHR system is critical to the success of the implementation of the PCEHR system.

(Developed from: Anderson, 2007; Xu and Quaddus, 2007; Xu and Quaddus, 2009; Vest, 2010; Xu and Quaddus, 2012; Xu et al., 2012; Xu et al., 2013; Pearce and Bainbridge, 2014; Xu et al., 2014; Partel, 2015; Cohen, 2016; Eden et al., 2016; Jawhari et al., 2016; Sherer et al., 2016; Brinkel et al., 2017)

Table-5 suggests individual factors that could have impact on adoption and use of the PCEHR system. Respondents need to indicate the extent to which they agree with the following statements where 1 indicates that they strongly disagree with the statement and 7 indicates they strongly agree with the statement.

Table-5 Individual differences

Individual Differences	Statements
Involvement	My involvement in the deployment of the PCEHR system would encourage the ownership and lead to the acceptance and use of the system.
Experience/Skill	My experience/skill in using new systems and new technologies will affect my acceptance and use of the PCEHR system. The more experienced I am, the more likely I would accept and use the system.
Personal Innovativeness	If I am innovative and would like to try new things, I would be more likely to accept and use the PCEHR system.
Computer Skills	I have sufficient computer skills, I would be more likely to accept and use the PCEHR system.
Attitude	If I don't feel comfortable and/or confident to manage and disseminate my health information electronically, I am less likely to accept and use the PCEHR system.

(Developed from Zmud, 1979; Brancheau and Wetherbe, 1990; Rogers, 1995; Gefen and Straub, 1997; Agarwal and Prasad, 1999; Agarwal and Prasad, 2000; Venkatesh and Davis, 2000; Xu and Quaddus, 2007; Aggelidis and Chatzoglou, 2009; Xu and Quaddus, 2009; Xu et al., 2012; Xu et al., 2013; Xu and Quaddus, 2007; Ludwick and Doucette, 2009; Xu and Quaddus, 2009; Xu and Quaddus, 2012; Xu *et al.*, 2012; Xu *et al.*, 2013; Nguyen *et al.*, 2014; Xu *et al.*, 2014; Sligo *et al.*, 2017)

Table-6 presents PCRHR system characteristics that have impact on adoption and use of the PCEHR system. Respondents need to indicate the extent to which they agree with the following statements where 1 indicates that they strongly disagree with the statement and 7 indicates they strongly agree with the statement.

Table-6 PCEHR system characteristics

PCEHR System Characteristics	Statements
Trialability	I should be able to try out the PCEHR system before I decide to use the system.
Accuracy, Completeness and Currency of the Information	Information in the PCEHR system should be accurate, complete, and current.
Access Control	I should be able to see all the activities in my PCEHR system accounts.
Information Control	I should have full control of my health/medical information in the PCEHR system.
Children Information Control	I should have full control of medical information of my children (especially those under the age of 14) in the PCEHR system.
Accessibility	I should be able to access my electronic health records in the PCEHR system anywhere and anytime via different computing devices and channels.

Availability	The PCEHR system should be available 24 hours, 365 days a year with very little and insignificant downtime.
Regional/District Integration	The PCEHR system should be integrated well with applications and systems of various health care providers across the region/district.
Cross-state Integration	The PCEHR system should be integrated well with applications and systems of various health care providers across the states.
Cross-border/International Integration	The PCEHR system should be integrated well with applications and systems of various healthcare providers outside Australia.
Maintenance and Updates	The PCEHR system should be maintained and updated regularly.
Delegation	The PCEHR system should allow me to delegate the management of my medical information in the system when necessary.

(Developed from Kwon and Zmud, 1987; Moore, 1987; Davis et al., 1992; Igbaria et al., 1995; Rogers, 1995; Agarwal and Prasad, 1997; Chau and Tam, 1997; Beatty et al., 2001; Hong et al., 2002; Xu and Quaddus, 2007; Xu and Quaddus, 2009; Xu and Quaddus, 2012; Xu et al., 2013; Xu and Quaddus, 2007; Ludwick and Doucette 2009; Xu and Quaddus, 2009; Xu and Quaddus, 2012; Xu et al., 2012; Xu et al., 2013; Jamoom et al., 2014; Kerai et al., 2014; Nguyen et al., 2014; Pearce and Bainbridge, 2014; Thurston, 2014; Xu et al., 2014; ; Partel, 2015; Barbarin et al., 2016; Chao, 2016; Eden et al., 2016; Jawhari et al. 2016; Palojoki et al., 2016; Sansom, 2016; Cunningham et al., 2017; Sligo et al., 2017; Swinn and Weber, 2017)

Table-7 lists statements regarding the perceived/expected benefits of the PCEHR system. Respondents need to indicate the extent to which they agree with the following statements where 1 indicates that they strongly disagree with the statement and 7 indicates they strongly agree with the statement.

Table-7 Perceived/expected benefits

Perceived/Expected Benefits	Statements
Personal Medical Information Management	The PCEHR system would help me better manage my personal medical information (especially electronically).
Better and New Services	The PCEHR system would help create better and new health services.
Efficiency/Productivity	The PCEHR system would help enhance the efficiency/productivity of health services.
Effectiveness	The PCEHR system would help improve the effectiveness of health services.
Quality	The PCEHR system would help improve the quality of

	health services.
Safety	The PCEHR system would help improve the safety of health services for Australian consumers.
Time and Cost Reduction	The PCEHR system would help reduce time & cost of health services.
Continuity of Health Services	The PCEHR system would ensure the continuity of health services for Australian consumers.
Health and Well-Being	The PCEHR system would improve my health/well-being.
Saving Lives	The PCEHR system would help save lives.
Equitable Access to Health Services	The PCEHR system would help provide equitable access to health services.
Continuity of Health Services	The PCEHR system would help improve the continuity of health services.

(Source: Developed from Xu and Quaddus, 2007; Xu and Quaddus, 2009; Xu and Quaddus, 2012; Xu et al., 2012; Xu et al., 2013; Jamoom et al., 2014; Nguyen et al., 2014; Thurston, 2014; Xu et al., 2014; Asan et al., 2016; Chao, 2016; Brinkel et al., 2017; Hoque and Sorwar, 2017; Swinn and Weber, 2017)

Table-8 includes statements regarding the perceived/expected user friendliness of the PCEHR system. Respondents need to indicate the extent to which they agree with the following statements where 1 indicates that they strongly disagree with the statement and 7 indicates they strongly agree with the statement.

Table-8 Perceived/expected user friendliness

Perceived/Expected User Friendliness	Statements
Simple to Learn and Use	The PCEHR system should be simple to learn and use with simple procedures.
Easy to Register	The PCEHR system should be easy to register.
Affordable to Learn and Use	The PCEHR system should be affordable to learn and use.
Speed	It should be fast to get the required information in the PCEHR system.
Easy to Contribute Information	It should be easy to contribute information in the system.
Privacy	The PCEHR system should effectively address the privacy concerns associated with using the system by establishing privacy policies and appropriate measures.
Security	The PCEHR system should effectively address the security concerns associated with using the system by establishing policies and appropriate measures.
Human Assistance and Interaction	I should be provided with the opportunities to communicate with customer service personnel when I

	encounter issues with the PCEHR system.
Multi-Channels Communication and Multiple Touch Points	I should be able to communicate with the operators of the PCEHR system via multiple channels and multiple touch points.
Communities	I should be provided with the opportunities to network with other users of the PCEHR system (online and offline).

(Developed from Anderson, 2007; Xu and Quaddus, 2007; Xu and Quaddus, 2009; Xu and Quaddus, 2012; Xu *et al.*, 2012; Xu *et al.*, 2013; Nguyen *et al.*, 2014; Xu *et al.*, 2014; Partel, 2015; Asan *et al.*, 2016; Barbarin *et al.*, 2016; Eden *et al.*, 2016; Jawhari *et al.*, 2016; Brinkel *et al.*, 2017; Hoque and Sorwar, 2017; Swinn and Weber, 2017).

Table-9 presents statements regarding the various influences on people's adoption and use of the PCEHR system. Respondents need to indicate the extent to which they agree with the following statements where 1 indicates that they strongly disagree with the statement and 7 indicates they strongly agree with the statement.

Table-9 Subject norms

Subject Norms	Statements
Peer Pressure/Influence	Peers have influence on my acceptance and use of the PCEHR system.
Following Early Users' Lead	I would follow earlier users' lead in accepting and using the PCEHR system.
Doctor's Lead	I would follow my doctors' lead in accepting and using the PCEHR system.
Respected People's Influence	I would accept and use the PCEHR system as a result of encouragement from respected people.
Doctor's Recommendation	I would accept and use the PCEHR system as a result of the recommendation from my doctors.
Media Influence	I would accept and use the PCEHR system as a result of the influence from the media.

(Developed from Thompson et al., 1991; Liker and Sindi, 1997; Lucas and Spitler, 1999, Xu and Quaddus, 2007; Aggelidis and Chatzoglou, 2009; Holden and Karsh, 2010; Cowan, 2016; Sansom, 2016; Swinn and Weber, 2017; Xu and Quaddus, 2007; Xu and Quaddus, 2009; Xu and Quaddus, 2012; Xu *et al.*, 2012; Xu *et al.*, 2013; Xu *et al.*, 2014; Asan *et al.*, 2016; Brinkel *et al.*, 2017; Hoque and Sorwar, 2017)

Table-10 consists of statements regarding the voluntary adoption and use of the PCEHR system. Respondents need to indicate the extent to which they agree with the following statements where 1 indicates that they strongly disagree with the statement and 7 indicates they strongly agree with the statement.

Table-10 Voluntariness

Voluntariness	Statements
Opt-in Model	The current opt-in model would make me feel comfortable to accept and use the PCEHR system.
Opt-out Model	The opt-out model would make me feel comfortable to accept and use the PCEHR system.
Mandatory Use	I should be required to use the PCEHR system for my health-related matters.
Linking to Benefits	Claims of government benefits & rebates should be linked to the PCEHR system.
Benefit Realization	I will use the PCEHR system when I see the benefits of using the system.

(Developed from Agarwal and Prasad, 1997; Bansler and Havn, 2002; Xu and Quaddus, 2007; Xu *et al.*, 2014; Pearce and Bainbridge, 2014; Partel, 2015; Coyne, 2017; Cunningham *et al.*, 2017; Swinn and Weber, 2017; Gribbin, 2018; Grubb, 2018; McCauley, 2018; Minion, 2018; Murphy, 2018)

Table-11 presents statements on adoption and use of the PCEHR system. Respondents need to indicate the extent to which they agree with the following statements where 1 indicates that they strongly disagree with the statement and 7 indicates they strongly agree with the statement.

Table-11 System adoption

Activities & Purposes of System Adoption	Statements
Uploading and Storing Information	I will use the PCEHR system for uploading and storing my medical information into the PCEHR system.
Disseminating and Sharing Information with Healthcare Providers	I will use the PCEHR system for disseminating and sharing my health/medical information with various healthcare providers.
Disseminating and Sharing Information with Government Agencies	I will use the PCEHR system for disseminating and sharing my health/medical information with government agencies.
Linking with Other Government Services	I will use the PCEHR system for linking the system with other services provided the government.
Managing Health Information	I will use the PCEHR system for using the system to manage my health/medical information.
Better Understanding of Health Conditions	I will use the PCEHR system for better understanding my health conditions and having better awareness of my health issues/concerns.

(Developed from Aggelidis and Chatzoglou, 2009; Bansler and Havn; Bhattacherjee, 2001; 2002; Holden and Karsh, 2010; Martins *et al.*, 2014; Xu and Quaddus, 2007; Xu and Quaddus, 2009; Xu and Quaddus, 2012; Xu *et al.*, 2012; Xu *et al.*, 2013; Jamoom *et al.*, 2014; Nguyen *et al.*, 2014; Xu *et al.*, 2014)

Table-12 lists statements regarding factors that would facilitate/encourage people's continued use of the PCEHR system. Respondents need to indicate the extent to which they agree with the following statements where 1 indicates that they strongly disagree with the statement and 7 indicates they strongly agree with the statement.

Table-12 Facilitating factors

Facilitating Factors	Statements
Incentives	Appropriate incentives (e.g., concessions and deductions) would encourage me to continue my use of the PCEHR system.
Imperatives	Appropriate imperatives (e.g., linking with payments and benefits from the government) would encourage me to continue my use of the PCEHR system.
Policy Updates	Appropriate policy updates regarding the use of PCEHR system would encourage me to continue my use of the PCEHR system.
System Improvements	Continuous system improvements (e.g., being easier for registration, accelerating introduction of more planned features (such as pathology and radiology results), being easier to contribute information, and increasing the range of information in the system) would encourage me to continue my use of the PCEHR system.
Promotion of Success Stories and Best Practices	Through promoting success stories and best practices of using the PCEHR system, I would be encouraged to continue my use of the system.
Promotion of Benefits	Through promoting benefits of using the PCEHR system, I would be encouraged to continue my use of the system.
Satisfying Needs Continuously	It should be ensured that the PCEHR system can continuously address my needs of health/medical information.
Encouragement	I should be encouraged to make the use of the PCEHR system a part of my life.
Good Governance	Good governance model of the PCEHR system would encourage me to continually use the system.
Funding	Sufficient and continuous funding for the PCEHR system should be provided by the government.
Better Training	Better training of using the system should be provided by the government.

(Developed from Ajzen and Fishbein, 1978; Rogers, 1985; Davis, 1986; Holden and Karsh, 2010; Anderson, 2007; Xu and Quaddus, 2007; Aggelidis and Chatzoglou, 2009; Xu and Quaddus, 2009; Xu and Quaddus, 2012; Xu et al., 2012; Xu et al., 2013; Jamoom et al., 2014; Pearce and Bainbridge, 2014; Xu et al., 2014; Partel, 2015; Cohen, 2016; Jawhari et al., 2016; Sansom, 2016; Sherer et al., 2016; Sligo et al., 2017; Swinn and Weber, 2017)

Table-13 lists statements regarding realized benefits of the PCEHR system. Respondents need to indicate the extent to which they agree with the following statements where 1 indicates that they strongly disagree with the statement and 7 indicates they strongly agree with the statement.

Table-13 Realized benefits

Realized Benefits	Statements
Personal Medical Information Management	The PCERH system has helped me better manage my personal medical information (especially electronically).
Better and New Services	The PCERH system has helped create better and new health services.
Efficiency/Productivity	The PCERH system has helped enhance the efficiency/productivity of health services.
Effectiveness	The PCERH system has helped improve the effectiveness of health services.
Quality	The PCERH system has helped improve the quality of health services.
Safety	The PCERH system has helped improve the safety of health services.
Time and Cost Reduction	The PCERH system has helped reduce time & cost of health services.
Continuity of Health Services	The PCERH system has helped ensure the continuity of health services.
Health and Well-Being	The PCERH system has helped improve my health/well-being.
Saving Lives	The PCERH system has helped save lives.
Equitable Access to Health Services	The PCERH system has helped provide equitable access to health services.
Continuity of Health Services	The PCERH system has helped improve the continuity of health services.

(Developed from Xu and Quaddus, 2007; Xu and Quaddus, 2009; Xu and Quaddus, 2012; Xu *et al.*, 2012; Xu *et al.*, 2013; Jamoom *et al.*, 2014; Nguyen *et al.*, 2014; Thurston, 2014; Xu *et al.*, 2014; Asan *et al.*, 2016; Chao, 2016; Brinkel *et al.*, 2017; Hoque and Sorwar, 2017; Swinn and Weber, 2017)

Table-14 lists statements regarding realized user friendliness of the PCEHR system. Respondents need to indicate the extent to which they agree with the following statements where 1 indicates that they strongly disagree with the statement and 7 indicates they strongly agree with the statement.

Table-14 Realized user friendliness

Realized User Friendliness	Statements
Simple to Learn and Use	The PCEHR system has demonstrated to be simple to learn and use with simple procedures.

Easy to Register	The PCEHR system has demonstrated to be easy to register. .
Affordable to Learn and Use	The PCEHR system has demonstrated to be affordable to learn and use with simple procedures.
Speed	It has demonstrated to be fast to get the required information in the PCEHR system.
Easy to Contribute Information	The PCEHR system has demonstrated to be easy to contribute information. .
Privacy	The PCEHR system has effectively demonstrated to be able to address the privacy concerns associated with using the system by establishing privacy policies and appropriate measures.
Security	The PCEHR system has demonstrated to be able to effectively address the security concerns associated with using the system by establishing policies and appropriate measures.
Human Assistance and Interaction	I have been provided with the opportunities to communicate with customer service personnel when I encounter issues with the PCEHR system.
Multi-Channels Communication and Multiple Touch Points	I have been able to communicate with the operators of the PCEHR system via multiple channels and multiple touch points.
Communities	I have been provided with the opportunities to network with other users of the PCEHR system (online and offline).

(Developed from Anderson, 2007; Xu and Quaddus, 2007; Xu and Quaddus, 2009; Xu and Quaddus, 2012; Xu *et al.*, 2012; Xu *et al.*, 2013; Nguyen *et al.*, 2014; Xu *et al.*, 2014; Partel, 2015; Asan *et al.*, 2016; Barbarin *et al.*, 2016; Eden *et al.*, 2016; Jawhari *et al.*, 2016; Brinkel *et al.*, 2017; Hoque and Sorwar, 2017; Swinn and Weber, 2017).

Table-15 displays statements regarding subject norms on continued use of the PCEHR system. Respondents need to indicate the extent to which they agree with the following statements where 1 indicates that they strongly disagree with the statement and 7 indicates they strongly agree with the statement.

Table-15 Subject norms on continued use

Subject Norms on Continued Use	Statements
Peer Pressure/Influence	Peers have influence on my continued use of the PCEHR system.
Following Early Users' Lead	I would follow earlier users' lead in continued use of the PCEHR system.
Doctor's Lead	I would follow my doctors' lead in continued use of the PCEHR system.

Respected People's Influence	I would continually use the PCEHR system as a result of encouragement from respected people.
Doctor's Recommendation	I would continually use the PCEHR system as a result of the recommendation from my doctors.
Media Influence	I would continually use the PCEHR system as a result of the influence from the media.

(Developed from Thompson et al., 1991; Liker and Sindi, 1997; Lucas and Spitler, 1999, Xu and Quaddus, 2007; Aggelidis and Chatzoglou, 2009; Holden and Karsh, 2010; Cowan, 2016; Sansom, 2016; Swinn and Weber, 2017; Xu and Quaddus, 2007; Xu and Quaddus, 2009; Xu and Quaddus, 2012; Xu *et al.*, 2012; Xu *et al.*, 2013; Xu *et al.*, 2014; Asan *et al.*, 2016; Brinkel *et al.*, 2017; Hoque and Sorwar, 2017)

Table-16 presents statements regarding the impact of voluntary use on people's continued use of the PCEHR system. Respondents need to indicate the extent to which they agree with the following statements where 1 indicates that they strongly disagree with the statement and 7 indicates they strongly agree with the statement.

Table-16 Voluntariness of continued use

Voluntariness of Continued Use	Statements
Opt-in Model	The current opt-in model would make me feel comfortable to continually use the PCEHR system.
Opt-out Model	The opt-out model would make me feel comfortable to continually use the PCEHR system.
Mandatory Use	I should be required to continually use the PCEHR system for my health related matters.
Linking to Benefits	Claims of government benefits & rebates should be continually linked to the PCEHR system.
Benefit Realization	I will continually use the PCEHR system when I have realized the benefits of using the system.

(Developed from Agarwal and Prasad, 1997; Bansler and Havn, 2002; Xu and Quaddus, 2007; Xu *et al.*, 2014; Pearce and Bainbridge, 2014; Partel, 2015; Coyne, 2017; Cunningham *et a*l., 2017; Swinn and Weber, 2017; Gribbin, 2018; Grubb, 2018; McCauley, 2018; Minion, 2018; Murphy, 2018)

Table-17 displays statements regarding continued use of the PCEHR system Respondents need to indicate the extent to which they agree with the following statements where 1 indicates that they strongly disagree with the statement and 7 indicates they strongly agree with the statement.

Table-17 Continued use

Continued Use	Statements
Uploading and Storing Information	I will continually use the PCEHR system for uploading and storing my medical information.
Disseminating and Sharing	I will continually use the PCEHR system for

Information with Healthcare Providers	disseminating and sharing my health/medical information with various healthcare providers.
Disseminating and Sharing Information with Government Agencies	I will continually use the PCEHR system for disseminating and sharing my health/medical information with government agencies.
Linking with Other Government Services	I will continually use the PCEHR system for linking the system with other services provided by the government.
Managing Health Information	I will continually use the PCEHR system for using the system to manage my health/medical information.
Better Understanding of Health Conditions	I will continually use the PCEHR system for better understanding my health conditions and having better awareness of my health issues/concerns.

(Developed from Aggelidis and Chatzoglou, 2009; Bansler and Havn, 2002; Bhattacherjee, 2001; Holden and Karsh, 2010; Martins *et al.*, 2014; Xu and Quaddus, 2007; Xu and Quaddus, 2009; Xu and Quaddus, 2012; Xu *et al.*, 2012; Xu *et al.*, 2013; Jamoom *et al.*, 2014; Nguyen *et al.*, 2014; Xu *et al.*, 2014)

3.3 Summary

A questionnaire of the PCEHR system adoption and continued use was discussed in detail in this chapter. Through going through various sections of the questionnaire, it can be seen that information of the PCEHR system users, their views & experiences on the implementation of the PCEHR system could be unveiled.

References

Agarwal, R. and Prasad, J. (1997), "The Role of Innovation Characteristics and Perceived Voluntariness in the Acceptance of Information Technologies", Decision Sciences, Vol. 28, No. 3, pp. 557-582.

Agarwal, R. and Prasad, J. (1999), "Are Individual Differences Germane to the Acceptance of New Information Technologies", Decision Sciences, Vol. 30, No. 2, pp. 361-391.

Agarwal , R. and Prasad, J. (2000), "A field study of the adoption of software process innovations by information systems professionals", IEEE Transaction on Engineering Management, Vol. 47, No. 3, pp. 295-308.

Aggelidis, V. P. and Chatzoglou, P. D. (2009), "Using a modified technology acceptance model in hospitals", International Journal of Medical Informatics, Vol. 78, pp.115-126.

Ajzen, I. and Fishbein, M. (1980), Understanding Attitudes and Predicting Social Behavior, Prentice-Hall, Inc., Englewood Cliffs, New Jersey 07632.

Anderson, J. G. (2007), "Social, ethical and legal barriers to E-health", International Journal of Medical Informatics, Vol. 76, pp.480-483.

Asan, O., Tyszka, J. and Fletcher, K. E. (2016), "Capturing the patient voices: Planning for patient-centered electronic health record use", International Journal of Medical Informatics, Vol. 95, pp.1-7. Australian Government (2017), Budget 2017-2018: Budget Statements 2017-18 Budget Related Paper No. 1.10, Health Portfolio, Online Available at: http://www.health.gov.au/internet/budget/publishing.nsf/Content/2017-2018_Health_PBS_sup4/$File/2017-18_Health_PBS_Complete.pdf (accessed on 14 May 2017).

Bansler, J.P. and Havn, E. (2002), "Exploring the role of networks in IT implementation-The case of knowledge management systems", The Xth European Conference on Information Systems, Gdansk, Poland, June 2002.

Barbarin, A. M., Klasnja, P. and Veinot, T. C. (2016), "Good or bad, ups and downs, and getting better: Use of personal health data for temporal reflection in chronic illness", International Journal of Medical Informatics, Vol. 94, pp. 237-245.

Beatty, R.C., Shim, J. P., and Jones, M.C. (2001), "Factors influencing corporate website adoption: a time-based assessment", Information & Management, Vol. 38, No. 6, pp. 337-354.

Bhattacherjee, A. (2001), "Understanding Information Systems Continuance: An Expectation-Confirmation Model", MIS Quarterly, Vol. 25, No. 3, pp. 351-370.

Brancheau, J. C. and Wetherbe, J. C. (1990), "The adoption of spreadsheet software: testing innovation diffusion theory in the context of end-user computing", Information Systems Research, Vol. 1, No. 2, pp. 123-139.

Brinkel, J., Dako-Gyeke, P., Kramer, A., May, J. and Fobil, J. N. (2017), "An investigation of user attitudes, requirements and willingness to use mobile phone-based interactive voice response systems for seeking healthcare in Ghana: A qualitative study", Public Health, Vol. 144, pp.125-133.

Chao, C. A. (2016), "The impact of electronic health records on collaborative work routines: A narrative network analysis", International Journal of Medical Informatics, Vol. 94, pp.100-111.

Chau, P. Y. K. and Tam, K. Y. (1997), "Factors affecting the adoption of open systems: An exploratory study", MIS Quarterly, Vol. 21, No. 1, pp. 1-24.

Cohen, M. F. (2016), "Impacts of the HIETH financial incentives on EHR adoption in small, physician-owned practices", International Journal of Medical Informatics, Vo. 94, pp.143-154.

Cowan, P. (2016), "Most Australian GP clinics aren't using e-health records", itnews, 6 April 2016, Online Available at: https://www.itnews.com.au/news/most-australian-gp-clinics-arent-using-e-health-records-417807 (accessed on 10 May 2017).

Coyne, A. (2017), "Budget 2017: Policy change backed by funding injection", itnews, 9 May 2017, Online Available at: https://www.itnews.com.au/news/every-australian-will-now-get-an-automatic-e-health-record-461072 (accessed on 9 May 2017).

Cunningham, C., Howson, J., Pearson, L. and Schofield, D. (2017), "Health navigator linking up the Wheatbelt through opt-out shared EHR", Pulse+IT, 3 April 2017, Online Available at: https://www.pulseitmagazine.com.au/australian-ehealth/3677-health-navigator-linking-up-the-wheatbelt-through-opt-out-shared-ehr (accessed on 4 April 2017).

Davis, F. D. (1986), A technology Acceptance Model for Empirically Testing New End-User Information Systems: Theory and Results, Doctoral Dissertation, Massachusetts Institute of Technology.

Davis, F. D., Bagozzi, R. P. and Warshaw, P. R. (1992), "Extrinsic and intrinsic motivation to use computers in the workplace", Journal of Applied Social Psychology, Vol. 22, No. 14, pp. 1111-1132.

Eden, K.B., Totten, A. M., Kassakian, S. Z., Gorman, P. N., McDonagh, M.S., Devine, B., Pappas, M., Daeges, M., Woods, S. and Hersh, W. R. (2016), "Barriers and facilitators to exchanging health information: A systematic review", International Journal of Medical Informatics, Vol. 88. pp. 44-51.

Gefen, D. and Straub, D. W. (1997), "Gender differences in the perceptions and use of E-mail: an extension to the technology acceptance model", MIS Quarterly, Vol. 21, No. 4, pp. 389-400.

Gribbin, C. (2018), "My Health Record: Greg Hunt bows to pressure, announces changes to address privacy concerns", ABC News, 1 August 2018, Online, Available at: http://www.abc.net.au/news/2018-07-31/court-order-needed-for-my-health-record-greg-hunt-says/10058544 (accessed on 1 August 2018).

Grubb, B. (2018), "Australians are 'rightly' questioning My Health Record, says Privacy Commissioner", The Sydney Morning Herald, 31 July 2018, Online, Available at: https://www.smh.com.au/technology/australians-are-rightly-questioning-my-health-record-says-privacy-commissioner-20180730-p4zui3.html (accessed on 1 August 2018).

Holden, R. J. and Karsh, B. T. (2010), "The Technology Acceptance Model: Its past and its future in health care", Journal of Biomedical Informatics, Vol. 43, pp.159-172.

Hong, W.Y., Thong, J. Y. L., Wong, W.W. and Tam, K. Y. (2002), "Determinants of user acceptance of digital libraries: an empirical examination of individual differences and system characteristics", Journal of Management Information Systems, Vol. 18, No. 3, pp. 97-124.

Hoque, R. & Sorwar, G. (2017), "Understanding factors influencing the adoption of mHealth by the elderly: An extension of the UTAUT model", International Journal of Medical Informatics, Vol. 101, pp.75-84.

Igbaria, M., Guimaraes, T. and Davis, G.B. (1995), "Testing the determinants of microcomputer usage via a structural equation model", Journal of Management Information Systems, Vol. 11, No. 4, pp. 87-114.

Jamoom, E. W., Patel, V., Furukawa, M. F. and King, J. (2014), "EHR adopters vs non-adopters: Impacts of, barriers to, and federal initiatives for EHR adoption", Healthcare, Vol. 2, pp. 33-39.

Jawhari, B., Keenan, L., Zakus, D., Ludwick, D., Isaac, A., Saleh, A. and Hayward, R. (2016), "Barriers and facilitators to Electronic Medical Record (EMR) use in an urban slum", International Journal of Medical Informatics, Vol. 94, pp.246-254.

Kerai, P., Wood, P. and Martin, M. (2014), "A pilot study on the views of elderly regional Australians of personally controlled electronic health records", International Journal of Medical Informatics, Vol. 83, pp. 201-209.

Kwon, T. H. and Zmud, R. W. (1987), "Unifying the fragment models of information systems implementation" in Critical Issues in Information System Research, eds R. J. Boland Jr. & R. A. Hirscheim, John Wiley & Sons, New York, pp. 227-251.

Lucas, H. C. and Spitler, V. K. (1999), "Technology use and performance: a field study of broker workstations", Decision Sciences, Vol. 30, No. 2, pp. 291-311.

Liker, J. K. and Sindi, A. A. (1997), "User acceptance of expert systems: A test of the theory of reasoned action", Journal of Engineering and Technology Management, Vol. 14, No. 2, pp. 147-173.

Ludwick, D. A. and Doucette, J. (2009), "Adopting electronic medical records in primary care: Lessons learned from health information systems implementation experience in seven countries", International Journal of Medical Informatics, Vol. 78, pp.22-31.

Martins, C., Oliveira, T. and Popovic, A. (2014), "Understanding the Internet banking adoption: A unified theory of acceptance and use of technology and perceived risk application", International Journal of Information Management, Vol. 34, pp.1-13.

McCauley, D. (2018), "Health Minister backs down on My Health Record", The Sydney Morning Herald, 31 July 2018, Online, Available at: https://www.smh.com.au/politics/federal/health-minister-backs-down-on-my-health-record-20180731-p4zuqo.html (accessed on 1 August 2018).

Minion, L. (2018), "Queensland threatens to disrupt My Health Record roll out with call for COAG to suspend opt out", Healthcare IT, 30 July 2018, Online, Available at: https://www.healthcareit.com.au/article/queensland-threatens-disrupt-my-health-record-roll-out-call-coag-suspend-opt-out (accessed on 1 August 2018).

Moore, G. C. (1987), "End-user computing and office automation: a diffusion of innovation perspectives', INFOR, Vol. 25, No. 3, pp. 214-235.

Muhammad, I., Teoh, S.Y. and Wickramasinghe, N. (2012), "The Application of a Sociotechnical Analysis for the Personally Controlled Electronic Health Record", In Proceedings of PACIS 2012.

Murphy, K. (2018), "My Health Record: Greg Hunt promises to redraft legislation after public outcry", The Guardian, 31 July 2018, Online, Available at: https://www.theguardian.com/australia-news/2018/jul/31/my-health-record-greg-hunt-promises-to-redraft-legislation-after-public-outcry (accessed on 1 August 2018).

My Health Record (2018), Opt out of My Health Record, Online, Available at: https://www.myhealthrecord.gov.au/for-you-your-family/opt-out-my-health-record (Accessed on 9 August 2018).

Nguyen, L., Bellucci, E. and Nguyen, L. T. (2014), "Electronic health records implementation: An evaluation of information system impact and contingency factor", International Journal of Medical Informatics, Vol. 83, pp. 779-796.

Palojoki, S., Pajunen, T. Saranto, K. and Lehtonen, L. (2016), "Electronic health record-related safety concerns: A cross-sectional survey of electronic health record users", JMIR Medical Informatics, Vol. 4, Issue 2, pp.1-12.

Partel, K. (2015), "Toward better implementation: Australia's My Health Record", Deeble Institute Issues Brief, No. 13, 30/10/2015, pp.1-20.

Pearce, C. and Bainbridge, M. (2014), "A personally controlled electronic health record for Australia", Journal of the American Medical Informatics Association, Vol. 21, pp.707-713.

Rogers, E. M. (1995), Diffusion of Innovations, Fourth Edition, The Free Press, New York, USA.

Sansom, M. (2016), "My Health Record: Medics speak up", Government News, 15 August 2016, Online Available at: http://www.governmentnews.com.au/2016/08/24703/ (accessed on 15 April 2017).

Sherer, S. A., Meyerhoefer, C. D. and Peng, L. (2016), "Applying institutional theory to the adoption of electronic health records in the U.S.", Information & Management, Vol. 53, pp.570-580.

Sligo, J., Gauld, R., Roberts, V. and Villa, L. (2017), "A literature review for large-scale health information system project planning, implementation and evaluation", International Journal of Medical Informatics, Vol. 97, pp.86-97.

Swinn, M. and Weber, M. (2017), "My Health Record: The resuscitation of e-health, or a data placebo?", Image & Data Manager, 13 April 2017, Online Available at: https://idm.net.au/article/0011469-my-health-record-resuscitation-e-health-or-data-placebo (accessed on 10 May 2017).

Thompson, R. L., Higgins, C. A. and Howell, J. M. (1991), "Personal computing: toward a conceptual model of utilization", MIS Quarterly, Vol. 15, No. 1, pp. 125-143.

Thurston, J. (2014), "Meaningful use of Electronic Health Records", The Journal of Nursing Practitioners, Vol. 10, Issue 7, pp. 510-513.

Venkatesh, V. and Davis, F. D. (2000), "A theoretical extension of the technology acceptance model: four longitudinal field studies", Management Science, Vol. 46, No. 2, pp. 186-204.

Xu, J. and Quaddus, M. (2007), "Exploring the Factors Influencing End Users' Acceptance of Knowledge Management Systems: Development of a Research Model of Adoption and Continued Use", Journal of Organizational and End-Users Computing, Vol. 19, No.4, pp. 57-79.

Xu. J. and Quaddus, M. (2009) ed., E-Business in the 21st Century: Realities, Challenges, and Outlook, World Scientific, Singapore.

Xu, J., Gao, X., and Sorwar, G. (2014), "A research model of consumers' adoption and continued use of the Personally Controlled Electronic Health Record (PCEHR) system", International Technology Management Review, Vol. 4, No.4, pp. 187-200.

Xu, J., Gao, X., Sorwar, G. and Croll, P. (2012), "Current Status, Challenges, and Outlook of E-Health Record Systems in Australia", 7th International Conference on Intelligence Systems and Knowledge Engineering, Dec 15-17, 2012, Beijing, China.

Xu, J., Gao, X., Sorwar, G. and Croll, P. (2013), "Implementation of E-Health Record Systems in Australia", International Technology Management Review, Vol. 3, No.2, pp. 92-104.

Zmud, R. W. (1979), "Individual differences and MIS success: a review of the empirical literature", Management Science, Vol. 25, No. 10, pp. 966-979.

Chapter 4

Australian Consumers' Perspectives of Personal Electronic Health Records

The chapter presents a study of surveying consumers/individual users in Australia by applying the survey questionnaire of PCEHR system adoption and continued use discussed in Chapter 3. The results of the survey suggest that while the consumers/individual users could use the system for storing and sharing their health information, they are deeply concerned about privacy and security perspectives of their health information in the system. And the results also suggest that health care providers (e.g., doctors) have significant impact on consumers in terms of adopting and using the PCEHR system.

Keywords: E-health record, PCEHR system, Views/perceptions, Acceptance and use, Individual users.

4.1 Introduction

In 2012, the implementation of a national personally controlled electronic health record (PCEHR) system (it was recently rebadged as My Health Record

(MyHR) system) started in Australia. This system allows doctors, hospitals and other healthcare providers to share individuals' health information to provide the best possible health care (Department of Health, 2016). So far more than AU$1 billion has been invested to deploy the PCEHR system and its associated infrastructure (Kerlin and Heath, 2014), the system has not been widely accepted by individuals. The implementation is still in its early stage (Review Panel, 2014), and more can be done to improve the system.

Meanwhile the interests of consumers have not been properly represented in the development and implementation of the PCEHR system. In the PCEHR review ordered by the Coalition Government, no review panel members represented consumers. In addition, there is a lack of empirical studies examining factors influencing the acceptance and continued use of the PCEHR system. This chapter aims to (1) address the gap in the literature through exploring individuals' perceptions/views of the PCEHR system by identifying factors or variables affecting the acceptance and the continued use of the PCEHR system having regard to the recommendations of the Review Panel (2014) and the findings by Xu et al., (2013) and factors and variables from the model by Xu et al., (2014); and (2) provide recommendations to deal with expectations of and issues perceived by individuals.

Staff and students of a university in Australia were invited to participate in an online questionnaire survey of the PCEHR system adoption and use, which was discussed in Chapter 3. Respondents were also encouraged to distribute the invitation to their friends, neighbours and others beyond the University. Two rounds of e-mail invitations were sent to two generic email lists of staff and students.

Frequency distribution is analysed and percentages are used to present the results. The results attempt to draw out major factors of enablers for and barriers to the acceptance and continued use of the PCEHR system. The higher the percentage of the respondents, the more important the factor is. In this research, a factor is considerably more important when the percentage is equal to or greater than 50%.

4.2 Feedback analysis

4.2.1 Survey participants

Completed survey questionnaires were examined closed, and only those questionnaires with all questions answered were accepted. The number of fully completed surveys totaled 66. Table-1 presents a summary of the demographic information.

Table-1 Summary of the respondents' demographic information

Demographics		Frequency	Percentage
Gender	Male	42	63.6%
	Female	24	36.4%
Age	60-65	7	10.6%
	50-59	17	25.8%
	40-49	15	24.2%
	30-39	13	19.7%
	18-29	6	9.1%
	<18 and >65	7	10.6%
State	New South Wales	49	74.2%
	Queensland	14	21.2%
	Victoria	3	4.6%
Education	Doctorate	11	16.7%
	Master	10	15.2%
	Graduate Certificate/Graduate Diploma	7	10.9%
	Honour	1	1.5%
	Bachelor	24	36.0%
	Others	13	19.7%
Occupation	Education professionals	19	28.8%
	Administrators	7	10.5%
	Managers	7	10.5%
	Technology/engineering professionals	6	9.0%
	Students	5	7.5%
	Healthcare professionals	4	6%
	Company directors/business owners	4	6%

	Accounting/consulting/legal professionals	3	4.5%
	Sales persons	2	3%
	Community and personal services workers	2	3%
	Tourism and hospitality staff	2	3%
	Public servant	1	1.5%
	Media professionals	1	1.5%
	Librarians	2	3%
Language	Native	50	75.8%
	Fluent in reading/speaking	16	24.2%
Weekly household income in 2014-2015	> $1800	14	21.2%
	$1501-$1800	13	19.7%
	$1101-$1500	9	13.6%
	$901-$1100	9	13.6%
	$701-$900	10	15.2%
	$401-$700	5	7.6%
	< $401	6	9.1%
Household composition	1 person	10	15.2%
	> 1 person	28	42.4%
	Including child(ren) under 14	15	22.7%
	Including member(s) above 65	7	10.6%
	Including members with chronic/mental health conditions or disabilities	5	7.6%
	Live in aged care home	1	1.5%
Aboriginal Australian or Torres Strait Islander		1	1.5%

It is noticed that people in the age range from 30 to 59 (69.7% of the respondents) seem more interested in the PCEHR system. The interest tends to go up with the increase in age. The largest cohort of survey respondents are educational professionals (28.8%), which could be the result of surveying staff and students in a university setting. 80.3% of the respondents have at least a Bachelor's degree, and tend to have more experience using the Internet and digital technologies and understanding system usability and other quality attributes more than other people.

Table-2 is a summary of registration status with the PCEHR system and experiences in using technology for healthcare. The respondents report varied e-health experience. 53% of the 66 respondents state they have had no e-health experience, 34.8% have experience in using electronic systems for healthcare supportive services (e.g., online appointment scheduling, checking in via kiosks, and claiming expense online), 15.2% have experience in participating in online health programs (e.g., health and fitness through diet and exercise programs), 13.6% have experience using telemedicine (e.g., enabling doctors and nurses to see and diagnose patients remotely), 9.1% have experience in online treatments and assessments, 18.2% have experience in using health-related phone/tablets apps, 24.2% have experience in using wearable health and fitness tracking technology, 1.5% gained e-health experience via registering with PCEHR system, and 1.5% have e-health research experience. For the majority of the respondents who have no e-health experience, understanding the benefits of the PCEHR system may lead to their acceptance of the system, however it is recognized that this could be a challenging task.

Table-2 Summary of PCEHR experience and e-health experience

Particulars		Frequency	Percentage
Sources to know the PCEHR system	Media	23	34.8%
	Other people	18	27.3%
	Healthcare providers	10	15.2%
	Promotion materials	10	15.2%
Engagement in PCEHR system implementation	Lack of detailed knowledge	45	68.2%
	Not engaged	49	74.2%
	Allowing all healthcare providers to access health records	51	77.3%
	Believing in PCEHR success	22	33.3%
E-health experience	none	35	53.0%
	Have used e-system(s)	23	34.8%
	Have used health apps	12	18.2%
	Have participated in e-health program(s)	10	15.2%
	Have used wearable technology for health	16	24.2%

	Have received online treatment/assessment	6	9.1%
	Have used tele-medicine	9	13.6%
	Have gained e-health experience via the PCEHR system	1	1.5%
	Have undertook e-health research	1	1.5%
PCEHR system registration	Have registered	7	10.6%
	Will register in the future	19	28.8%
	Have registered for more than 12 and less than 24 months	6	9.1%
	Have registered for 24 months or longer	1	1.5%
	Registered without other's assistance	5	7.6%
	Registered with other's assistance	2	3.0%
	Registered on the Web	4	6.1%
	Registered in clinics	1	1.5%
	Registered at a mobile station/booth	1	1.5%
	Registered in offices of other healthcare providers	1	1.5%
	Have never used the system since registration	4	6.1%

Some important sources for survey respondents to become aware of the PCEHR systems include (in order): from the media (including TV, website, radio, newspaper, magazine, or other media Channels) (34.8% of the 66 respondents); from other people (e.g., my friends, my family members, colleagues, neighbours or people I met/talked to) (27.3%); from healthcare providers (15.2%); and from promotion materials received from governments and/or their agencies (15.2%). The majority of the survey respondents (68.2%) lack knowledge of the PCEHR system, and either have no knowledge/understanding of the PCEHR system or don't know much about the system. 74.2% of the respondents have not been involved in the implementation/roll-out of the PCEHR system, and 77.3% are happy to let health care providers (other than their GP) access (either on a regular basis or case-by-case manner) their medical information in the system (either full access or partial access). Meanwhile only 33.3% of the survey respondents believe the PCEHR system will be successful in the future.

Among the 66 survey respondents, only 7 (10.6%) have registered for the system (including registration of their dependent children) while another 19 (28.8%) suggest that they will register with the system in the future. Among the 7 respondents who have registered, 6 have been registered for between 12 and 24 months, and one has been registered for more than 24 months. In addition, the majority (57.1%) of the 7 registered respondents have not used the system at all after their registration with the system (either don't want to use or don't know how to use).

4.2.2 Factors affecting decision on acceptance/adoption

Table-3 shows a number of external factors and influences that affect users' perceptions of the PCEHR system, which in turn influences their acceptance and use of the system. This study identifies the importance of these factors corresponding to the percentage of respondents who rated that importance. The higher the percentage of the respondents, the more important the factor is. It is noted that a factor is considered 'important' when the percentage is greater than 50%.

Table-3 External Factors and Influences

External Factors & Influences	Questionnaire Items	Percentage of Respondents
Regulations and Policies	The regulations and policies relevant to the PCEHR system (e.g., Healthcare Identifiers Act 2010, Personally Controlled Electronic Health Records Act 2012) are essential to the implementation of the PCEHR system.	72.7%
ICT Infrastructure Development	The deployment of national broadband and investments in e-heath infrastructure by federal and state governments have laid the foundation for the implementation of the PCEHR system.	56.1%
Mobility	The increasing mobility of population from one place to another needs the PCEHR system so I can access my health information anywhere.	84.8%
Availability of Computing Equipment and Popularity of Mobile Devices	The wide availability of computing equipment and the popularity of mobile devices have made the PCEHR system more popular.	71.2%
Affordability and Accessibility of Internet Services	The high Internet penetration in Australia (more than 85%), as a result of good nationwide technology infrastructure and affordability, has	63.6%

	made the PCEHR system more appealing.	
Economic Uncertainty	The uncertainty of Australian economy will have impact on the future development of the PCEHR system.	43.9%
Continuity of the Government	The instability of Federal and State governments will have an impact on the implementation of the PCEHR system.,	59.1%
Unified Approach	Australia's multi-tier government system and large private sector has made the implementation of the PCEHR system extremely complex.	65.2%
Transparency and Communication of The Operations of the PCEHR System	Improved transparency and communication regarding the operations of the PCEHR system could have positive impact on the implementation of the system.	87.9%
Governance	Good governance model of the PCEHR system is critical to the success of the implementation of the PCEHR system.	89.4%

It can be seen that most of the external factors and influences are perceived to be important by the respondents. However, the importance of economic uncertainty is not supported by the respondents. This implies that the majority of the respondents (56.1%) believe that once the PCEHR system is fully operational, the system will remain in place despite any change of government and that for the greater good of the community, it is imperative to allocate sufficient IT resources and infrastructure for the continuity of the system.

Implementation of the PCEHR system largely depends on governance (89.4%). In addition to effective governance, other important government initiatives include: ensuring transparency and communications of the operations of the system (87.9%) and developing and implementing regulations and policies for the PCEHR system (72.7%).

By way of background, Australia has had two governments since the first release of the PCEHR system in 2012. Continuity of government is viewed as important to the implementation of the PCEHR system although some regulations and policies changed in 2014 after a review of the system was undertaken. 65.2% of the respondents believe Australia's multi-tier government system and large private sector does not make implementation of the PCEHR system easy. The PCEHR system is a national system, and the Medicare policy is applicable to all Australian residents, however state governments are expected to play an important role in the implementation. State/territory governments are expected to contribute to the funding of the PCEHR system (cited in the Consumers Health Forum of Australia, 2011) as well as the private sector (e.g., private hospitals and clinics, insurance firms). Other important external factors include: the increasing population mobility (84.8%), the wide availability of end-user computing equipment and the popularity of consumer mobile devices (71.2%), the affordable and accessible Internet services in Australia (63.6%), and the developed ICT infrastructure for e-health (56.1%).

Table-4 Individual differences

Individual Differences	Questionnaire Items	Percentage of Respondents
Involvement	My involvement in the deployment of the PCEHR system would encourage the ownership and lead to the acceptance and use of the system.	42.4%
Experience/Skill	My experience/skill in using new systems and new technologies will affect my acceptance and use of the PCEHR system. The more experienced I am, the more likely I would accept and use the system.	77.3%
Personal Innovativeness	If I am innovative and would like to try new things, I would be more likely to accept and use the PCEHR system.	68.2%
Computer Skills	I have sufficient computer skills, I would be more likely to accept and use the PCEHR system.	75.8%
Attitude	If I don't feel comfortable and/or confident to manage and disseminate my health information electronically, I am less likely to accept and use the PCEHR system.	68.2%

Table-4 examines individual differences that may be important to survey respondents' decision regarding acceptance and use of the PCEHR system which includes: general computer skills (75.8%), experience in using new systems (77.3%), personal innovativeness (68.2%) and attitude towards managing personal health information (68.2%). It is evident that the individual's involvement in the deployment of the PCEHR system is not viewed as important by the respondents. One possible explanation is the lack of experience in becoming involved with the system deployment (i.e., as reported in the previous Section of Demographic information wherein 74.2% of the respondents have not been involved in the implementation/roll-out of the PCEHR system). This could lead to the respondents' unawareness of the importance and benefits of users' involvement in the system development and implementation. On the other hand, some users could have the view that the government should play the key role in the system deployment since it is a government initiative and project.

Table-5 PCEHR system characteristics

PCEHR System Characteristics	Questionnaire Items	Percentage of Respondents
Trialability	I should be able to try out the PCEHR system before I decide to use the system.	89.4%
Accuracy, Completeness and Currency of the Information	Information in the PCEHR system should be accurate, complete, and current.	93.9%
Access Control	I should be able to see all the activities in my PCEHR system accounts.	97%
Information Control	I should have full control of my health/medical information in the PCEHR system.	90.9%
Children Information Control	I should have full control of medical information of my children (especially those under the age of 14) in the PCEHR system.	87.9%
Accessibility	I should be able to access my electronic health records in the PCEHR system anywhere and anytime via different computing devices and channels.	92.4%
Availability	The PCEHR system should be available 24 hours, 365 days a year with very little and insignificant downtime.	93.9%
Regional/District Integration	The PCEHR system should be integrated well with applications and systems of various health care providers across the region/district.	93.9%
Cross-state Integration	The PCEHR system should be integrated well with applications and systems of various health care providers across the states.	92.4%
Cross-border/International Integration	The PCEHR system should be integrated well with applications and systems of various healthcare providers outside Australia.	66.7%
Maintenance and Updates	The PCEHR system should be maintained and updated regularly.	93.9%
Delegation	The PCEHR system should allow me to	89.4%

	delegate the management of my medical information in the system when necessary.	

As seen in Table-5, all the characteristics of the PCEHR system are viewed by respondents as important, including data quality, accessibility/ubiquity, availability, interoperability/regional/district integration, maintenance/updates, trialability, access control, information control, children information control, and delegation. More particularly, the largest percentage (97%) are concerned with access control i.e., respondents should be able to see all the information contained in their health record.

Table-6 Perceived/expected benefits

Perceived/Expected Benefits	Questionnaire Items	Percentage of Respondents
Personal Medical Information Management	The PCEHR system would help me better manage my personal medical information (especially electronically).	89.9%
Better and New Services	The PCEHR system would help create better and new health services.	78.8%
Efficiency/Productivity	The PCEHR system would help enhance the efficiency/productivity of health services.	87.9%
Effectiveness	The PCEHR system would help improve the effectiveness of health services.	87.9%
Quality	The PCEHR system would help improve the quality of health services.	78.8%
Safety	The PCEHR system would help improve the safety of health services for Australian consumers.	81.8%
Time and Cost Reduction	The PCEHR system would help reduce time & cost of health services.	83.3%
Continuity of Health Services	The PCEHR system would ensure the continuity of health services for Australian consumers.	84.8%
Health and Well-Being	The PCEHR system would improve my health/well-being.	62.1%
Saving Lives	The PCEHR system would help save lives.	77.3%
Equitable Access to Health Services	The PCEHR system would help provide equitable access to health services.	65.2%
Continuity of Health	The PCEHR system would help improve the	83.3%

Services	continuity of health services.	

As seen in Table-6, most respondents share the views of the Review Panel (2014) regarding the values of the PCEHR system (e.g., efficiency, effectiveness, quality, safety, cost reduction, continuity of health services and saving lives). Moreover, other expected benefits of the system include: better management of personal medical information (89.9% of the respondents), better and new services (78.8%), provision of equitable access to health services (65.2%), and improved health and well-being (62.1%).

Table-7 Perceived/expected user friendliness

Perceived/Expected User Friendlincss	Questionnaire Items	Percentage of Respondents
Simple to Learn and Use	The PCEHR system should be simple to learn and use with simple procedures.	93.9%
Easy to Register	The PCEHR system should be easy to register.	92.4%
Affordable to Learn and Use	The PCEHR system should be affordable to learn and use.	92.4%
Speed	It should be fast to get the required information in the PCEHR system.	90.9%
Easy to Contribute Information	It should be easy to contribute information in the system.	90.9%
Privacy	The PCEHR system should effectively address the privacy concerns associated with using the system by establishing privacy policies and appropriate measures.	95.5%
Security	The PCEHR system should effectively address the security concerns associated with using the system by establishing policies and appropriate measures.	98.5%
Human Assistance and Interaction	I should be provided with the opportunities to communicate with customer service personnel when I encounter issues with the PCEHR system.	93.9%
Multi-Channels Communication and Multiple Touch Points	I should be able to communicate with the operators of the PCEHR system via multiple channels and multiple touch points.	90.9%
Communities	I should be provided with the opportunities to network with other users of the PCEHR	50%

	system (online and offline).	

As reflected in Table-7, respondents value the usability of the PCEHR system in terms of being simple to learn and use; easy to register; affordable to learn and use; easy to contribute information; and fast performance/speed. The respondents also expect user support in terms of human assistance and interaction, and multichannel communication and multi touch points. Respondents' most serious concerns associated with the PCEHR system are privacy (95.5%) and security (98.5%). Interestingly, 50% of the respondents don't think it necessary to have social communities of PCEHR system users. One possible explanation may be that they may not be willing to discuss their confidential personal medical information with strangers in a community i.e., they may only trust their doctors and respected people.

Table-8 Subject norms

Subject Norms	Questionnaire Items	Percentage of Respondents
Peer Pressure/Influence	Peers have influence on my acceptance and use of the PCEHR system.	36.4%
Following Early Users' Lead	I would follow earlier users' lead in accepting and using the PCEHR system.	34.8%
Doctor's Lead	I would follow my doctors' lead in accepting and using the PCEHR system.	69.7%
Respected People's Influence	I would accept and use the PCEHR system as a result of encouragement from respected people.	57.6%
Doctor's Recommendation	I would accept and use the PCEHR system as a result of the recommendation from my doctors.	72.7%
Media Influence	I would accept and use the PCEHR system as a result of the influence from the media.	25.8%

Table-8 suggests that while the respondents will follow and listen to their doctor and respected people regarding adoption and use of the PCEHR system, they believe in doctors' recommendation (72.7%) and guidance (69.7%) more than respected people (57.6%) regarding registration and acceptance. Respondents tend NOT to follow peers (100% - 36.4% = 63.6%) or early users (100% - 34.8% = 65.2%), and many people may not follow media promotions (100% - 25.8% = 74.2%). One possible explanation may be that when discussing medical matters, people only trust their doctor and other respected people since such matters are personal and could involve sensitive information.

Table-9 Voluntariness

Voluntariness	Questionnaire Items	Percentage of Respondents
Opt-in Model	The current opt-in model would make me feel comfortable to accept and use the PCEHR system.	68.2%
Opt-out Model	The opt-out model would make me feel comfortable to accept and use the PCEHR system.	57.6%
Mandatory Use	I should be required to use the PCEHR system for my health-related matters.	37.8%
Linking to Benefits	Claims of government benefits & rebates should be linked to the PCEHR system.	74.2%
Benefit Realization	I will use the PCEHR system when I see the benefits of using the system.	84.8%

Table-9 suggests that the opt-in policy (68.2%) is preferred over the opt-out policy (57.6%), although both are acceptable. The key motivating factors are benefit considerations, including linking government benefits to the PCHER system (74.2%) and the benefits realised by individuals (84.8%). Mandatory use may work, but will not work well as many individuals (100% -37.8% = 62.2%) do not feel comfortable with its use.

Table-10 System adoption

System Adoption	Questionnaire Items	Percentage of Respondents
Uploading and Storing Information	I will use the system for uploading and storing my medical information into the PCEHR system.	83.3%
Disseminating and Sharing Information with Healthcare Providers	I will use the system for disseminating and sharing my health/medical information with various healthcare providers.	83.3%
Disseminating and Sharing Information with Government Agencies	I will use the system for disseminating and sharing my health/medical information with government agencies.	48.5%
Linking with Other Government Services	I will use the system for linking the system with other services provided the government.	48.5%
Managing Health	I will use the system for using the system to	81.5%

Information	manage my health/medical information.	
Better Understanding of Health Conditions	I will use the system for better understanding my health conditions and having better awareness of my health issues/concerns.	69.7%

It can be deduced from Table-10 that more than 80% of the respondents will transfer their health data from current systems to the PCEHR system (uploading and storing information) to manage the data and more importantly to share the data with healthcare providers. Only 48.5% of respondents anticipate using the system for other purposes such as sharing information with government agencies or linking with other government services. Survey respondents may be afraid that their medical information will be inappropriately used for purposes other than medical matters (e.g., for insurance-related matters, for employment-related concerns). Respondents also expect that they can understand and monitor their own health condition better (69.7%) by accessing their personal health data.

4.2.3 Factors affecting consumers' decision of continued use

Table-11 Facilitating factors

Facilitating Factors	Questionnaire Items	Percentage of Respondents
Incentives	Appropriate incentives (e.g., concessions and deductions) would encourage me to continue my use of the PCEHR system.	62.1%
Imperatives	Appropriate imperatives (e.g., linking with payments and benefits from the government) would encourage me to continue my use of the PCEHR system.	62.1%
Policy Updates	Appropriate policy updates regarding the use of PCEHR system would encourage me to continue my use of the PCEHR system.	68.2%
System Improvements	Continuous system improvements (e.g., being easier for registration, accelerating introduction of more planned features (such as pathology and radiology results), being easier to contribute information, and increasing the range of information in the system) would encourage me to continue my use of the PCEHR system.	84.8%
Promotion of Success Stories and Best Practices	Through promoting success stories and best practices of using the PCEHR system, I would be encouraged to continue my use of the system.	66.7%

Promotion of Benefits	Through promoting benefits of using the PCEHR system, I would be encouraged to continue my use of the system.	68.2%
Satisfying Needs Continuously	It should be ensured that the PCEHR system can continuously address my needs of health/medical information.	83.3%
Encouragement	I should be encouraged to make the use of the PCEHR system a part of my life.	54.5%
Good Governance	Good governance model of the PCEHR system would encourage me to continually use the system.	77.3%
Funding	Sufficient and continuous funding for the PCEHR system should be provided by the government.	89.4%
Better Training	Better training of using the system should be provided by the government.	78.8%

As seen in Table-11, respondents believe that to induce users' continued use of the PCEHR system, it needs to continuously provide better services (84.8% of the respondents) and continuous funding for system improvements from the government (89.4%) since the PCEHR system is an expensive project. Among other factors influencing users' decision regarding continued use of the PCEHR system, user training (78.8%) and governance (77.3%) are viewed as more important than policy updates (68.2%), promotion of benefits (68.2%) awareness of success stories (66.7%), incentives (62.1%) or imperatives (62.1%), and other encouragement (54.5%).

Table-12 Realized benefits

Realized Benefits	Questionnaire Items	Percentage of Respondents
Personal Medical Information Management	I will continually use the system if it has helped me better manage my personal medical information (especially electronically).	87.9%
Better and New Services	I will continually use the system if it has helped create better and new health services.	83.3%
Efficiency/Productivity	I will continually use the system, if it has helped enhance the efficiency/productivity of health services.	84.8%
Effectiveness	I will continually use the system if it has helped improve the effectiveness of health services.	86.4%

Quality	I will continually use the system if it has helped improve the quality of health services.	83.3%
Safety	I will continually use the system if it has helped improve the safety of health services.	89.4%
Time and Cost Reduction	I will continually use the system, if it has helped reduce time & cost of health services.	87.8%
Continuity of Health Services	I will continually use the system if it has helped ensure the continuity of health services.	89.4%
Health and Well-Being	I will continually use the system, if it has helped improve my health/well-being.	81.8%
Saving Lives	I will continually use the system if it has helped save lives.	83.3%
Equitable Access to Health Services	I will continually use the system if it has helped provide equitable access to health services.	86.4%
Continuity of Health Services	I will continually use the system if it has helped improve the continuity of health services.	86.4%

Table-12 highlights that on average about 85% of respondents agree that realized benefits arising from using the PCEHR system are important to their decision of continuously using the system.

Table-13 Realized user friendliness

Realized User Friendliness	Questionnaire Items	Percentage of Respondents
Simple to Learn and Use	I will continually use the system if the PCEHR system has demonstrated to be simple to learn and use with simple procedures.	75.8%
Easy to Register	I will continually use the system if the PCEHR system has demonstrated to be easy to register.	74.2%
Affordable to Learn and Use	I will continually use the system if the PCEHR system has demonstrated to be affordable to learn and use with simple procedures.	75.8%
Speed	I will continually use the system if it has demonstrated to be fast to get the required information in the PCEHR system.	74.2%
Easy to Contribute	I will continually use the system, if the PCEHR	75.8%

Information	system has demonstrated to be easy to contribute information. .	
Privacy	I will continually use the system if the PCEHR system has effectively demonstrated to be able to address the privacy concerns associated with using the system by establishing privacy policies and appropriate measures.	78.8%
Security	I will continually use the system if the PCEHR system has demonstrated to be able to effectively address the security concerns associated with using the system by establishing policies and appropriate measures.	78.8%
Human Assistance and Interaction	I will continually use the system if I have been provided with the opportunities to communicate with customer service personnel when I encounter issues with the PCEHR system.	75.8%
Multi-Channels Communication and Multiple Touch Points	I will continually use the system if I have been able to communicate with the operators of the PCEHR system via multiple channels and multiple touch points.	71.2%
Communities	I will continually use the system if I have been provided with the opportunities to network with other users of the PCEHR system (online and offline).	37.9%

As indicated in Table-13, all the variables of realized user friendliness of the PCEHR system are viewed as important by the respondents regarding their decision to continually use the system. Similar to previously discussed factors of perceived user friendliness, the only exception is community variable, which only receives 37.9% agreement from the respondents. This further reinforces the concept that users are never willing to discuss their confidential personal medical information with other users, and that they only trust their doctors and respected people.

Table-14 Subject norms on continued use

Subject Norms on Continued Use	Questionnaire Items	Percentage of Respondents
Peer Pressure/Influence	Peers have influence on my continued use of the PCEHR system.	31.8%
Following Early Users' Lead	I would follow earlier users' lead in continued use of the PCEHR system.	39.4%

Doctor's Lead	I would follow my doctors' lead in continued use of the PCEHR system.	68.2%
Respected People's Influence	I would continually use the PCEHR system as a result of encouragement from respected people.	50%
Doctor's Recommendation	I would continually use the PCEHR system as a result of the recommendation from my doctors.	71.2%
Media Influence	I would continually use the PCEHR system as a result of the influence from the media.	28.8%

Compared to Table-8, Table-14 indicates that the respondents regard the subject norm as the same for both acceptance and continued use of the PCEHR system. In other words, while the respondents will follow and listen to their doctor and respected people regarding continued use of the PCEHR system, they will not be influenced by peers, early users of the system, or the media.

Table-15 Voluntariness of continued use

Voluntariness of Continued Use	Questionnaire Items	Percentage of Respondents
Opt-in Model	The current opt-in model would make me feel comfortable to continually use the PCEHR system.	71.2%
Opt-out Model	The opt-out model would make me feel comfortable to continually use the PCEHR system.	53%
Mandatory Use	I should be required to continually use the PCEHR system for my health related matters.	37.8%
Linking to Benefits	Claims of government benefits & rebates should be continually linked to the PCEHR system.	66.7%
Benefit Realization	I will continually use the PCEHR system when I have realized the benefits of using the system.	77.3%

Compared to Table-9, Table-15 indicates that the majority of the respondents believe both the use and continued use of the PCEHR system should not be mandatory even though they have different views on the opt-in and opt-out approaches, and the benefit considerations (including linking government benefits with the PCHER system and the benefits realised by individuals) are important for decisions regarding both the use and continued use of the system.

Table-16 Continued use

Continued Use	Questionnaire Items	Percentage of Respondents
Uploading and Storing Information	I will continually use the system for uploading and storing my medical information into the PCEHR system.	84.8%
Disseminating and Sharing Information with Healthcare Providers	I will continually use the system for disseminating and sharing my health/medical information with various healthcare providers.	80.3%
Disseminating and Sharing Information with Government Agencies	I will continually use the system for disseminating and sharing my health/medical information with government agencies.	45.5%
Linking with Other Government Services	I will continually use the system for linking the system with other services provided by the government.	57.6%
Managing Health Information	I will continually use the system for using the system to manage my health/medical information.	86.4%
Better Understanding of Health Conditions	I will continually use the system for better understanding my health conditions and having better awareness of my health issues/concerns.	75.8%

Compared to Table-10, Table-16 indicates that the respondents remain consistent in terms of the use and continuous use the PCEHR system. One minor difference is that while 57.6% of the respondents are in favour of linking the PCEHR system with other government services which could encourage their initial decision of adopting and using the PCEHR system, a slightly lower percentage of the respondents (48.5%) would view such activities & purposes could also have impact on their decision of continued use of the system. Given the small sample size, it could be argued that they are in the same range.

4.3 Discussion

The opt-out policy would register all eligible Australian residents in the PCEHR system however there is a long way to go to gain the acceptance and continued use of the system, especially from individual users. Acceptance and continued use needs the efforts of all stakeholders to resolve the issues of governance, meaningful use of the system, transparency, privacy, system security, quality and usability, education and promotion of the system's benefits.

Registration

Since the first release of the PCEHR system in July 2012, only a small percentage of Australian residents have voluntarily registered themselves with the system under the opt-in policy. The opt-in policy was not effective towards acceptance of the system by individuals. In 2014, the opt-out policy commenced as a pilot to automatically register eligible individual. The automatic registration meets the high expectation of ease of registration. However, registration is only a prerequisite for acceptance. Individuals tend to make a decision on acceptance of the system according to their doctors' recommendation and/or guidance. It is recommended that government should distribute promotion materials through doctors and provide bonuses for doctors' efforts in the recommendation and/or guidance according to completed registrations to the PCEHR system, as was the case in China (Gao et al., 2013). Health data may be critical to lives, and will be used mainly by healthcare providers. The influence of non-professional individuals on the registration decision is limited. Online forums by healthcare professionals may be helpful. Brochures and/or posters placed in clinics, hospitals and other places of healthcare services can be more effective than information on websites such as Medicare. Traditional forms of promotion used in commerce, such as media and word-of-mouth, may not be effective.

Many (if not most) doctors in Australia lack confidence in the PCEHR system for concerns such as risk, liability, insurance, security and information currency. Logically convincing and enticing doctors and other healthcare providers to use and promote the PCEHR system is critical to recommendation/advice from them. Patient registration with the PCEHR system as a condition of accreditation of a medical practice does not engender support for the PCEHR system by doctors.

Privacy and security

The current release of the PCEHR system is far from mature and suffers criticisms from major stakeholders. From individuals' perspectives, information privacy and data security are major concerns that affect individuals' decisions regarding acceptance and continued use of the PCEHR system. The privacy issue is directed towards access by users and the extended usage of the health records. Individuals would expect that they themselves manage their medical records and over time better understand their health conditions while health care providers utilize such information for healthcare services. Individuals are not comfortable if their records are used by other users or for other purposes. Therefore it is recommended that (1) the government should develop a policy of meaningful use of the PCEHR system that determines which authorised users access the right data for the correct purposes in the right circumstances, and (2) the integration and consolidation advice from healthcare providers, legal workers, system operators and other possible users. The policy should ensure the PCEHR system is used effectively without violating individuals' privacy in terms of the Privacy Act 1988.

Security should be a technical issue. System developers, together with healthcare providers and individuals, should identify threats to health data security, conduct risk analysis, and provide technical solutions to the threats. The solution should ensure appropriate secrecy, integrity and necessity (Schneider, 2015) so that sensitive data are unintelligible by unauthorised people or organisations, critical data cannot be changed by unauthorised people or organisations, and vital data in emergency situations are instantly accessible. Policy on security is important as well. A document in plain English about the security should be issued by the government. Online live chat forums or pop-up assistants (which are expected by individuals), should be available to answer questions about privacy, security and other issues.

Currently the MyGov portal links various government services, including the PCEHR system (it is called My Health Record now) (Department of Health, 2016) and different government agencies. It is not transparent in terms of the use of data among different services. It is recommended that the operator of MyGov should clearly describe and explain the use of all data collected in the system.

Benefits and technology

Individuals expect all the benefits from the PCEHR project as outlined by the Review Panel (2014), while many individuals do not wish to integrate the PCEHR system with other services, especially government services, as well as commercial and financial services. This attitude largely limits the benefits for individuals and, in turn, affects the acceptance of the system. Apart from the benefits that will accrue to individuals, the PCEHR system will also bring social benefits. Currently individuals are defined as consumers (Australian Government, 2012). Based on this definition, individuals do not expect the use of the PCEHR system to be made mandatory. This definition is a barrier to the acceptance and use of the system. It is recommended that individuals are defined as 'citizens' with respect to the PCEHR system. While enjoying privileges, a citizen must also comply with legal requirements. Information should highlight savings that will result from using the system, whilst in contrast, not using the system will require more welfare. Australia may introduce a 'PCEHR Levy', which may be additional to the Medicare Levy or similar to the Flood Levy imposed in 2011 and 2012 (Australian Taxation Office, 2015).

The Internet of Things (Gubbi et al., 2013) changes traditional concepts and improves people's life. For example, a smart phone is not only a telephone but also a computer, a GPS, a wallet, and a portable hand-held device containing apps used in everyday life. For healthcare purposes, a smart phone can be used for information and time management, health record maintenance and access, communications and consulting, reference and information gathering, patient management and monitoring, clinical decision-making, and medical education and training. More importantly, it can access point-of-care tools (Ventola, 2014). The Industry 4.0 upsurged from Germany (Brettel et al., 2014) introduces the concept of 'smart' process control. The PCEHR system, as a 'Thing' on the Internet, will bring unpredictable benefits for individuals, as a smart phone currently does. The system developers should design the system in such a way that it can use and be used by other 'Things'. The policy of meaningful use should also take the concepts of smart Things and smart processes into account.

System usability and quality attributes

Individuals do not intend to be involved in system development, but expect usability. It is recommended that system developers should interview a sample of the main users (individuals and healthcare providers) to understand their human and technical aspects for using the system. Different interface versions may be needed for different users according to such factors as: users' roles in the system, their age, their approaches and ways of accessing health records, their computing skills and Internet usage, and their health conditions. Some users may need special aids.

Individuals are also interested in other system characteristics including data quality, system ubiquity, interoperability, availability, testability and maintainability. System developers should document these quality attributes in plain English. Aspects dealing with delegation and access/information control should be addressed by meaningful use (policy) and privilege control (technology).

4.4 Summary

This chapter makes contribution to the literature by providing understanding of expectations and issues of the PCEHR system perceived by Australian consumers and by presenting practical recommendations/solutions to deal with their perceived expectations and issues.

The results of the research reported in this chapter could assist Australian government and other stakeholders (e.g., healthcare providers, legal professionals, PCEHR system developers, and others) in understanding the current status and challenges/issues associated with the implementation of the PCEHR system among Australian consumers and contribute to the development of practical guidelines to assist in that implementation. The results of this study could also offer some insights and recommendations for improving the government's efforts in deploying the PCEHR system and increasing the efficiency of resources required for the implementation. One major limitation of this study is the sample size not being large enough for research on the national system. Future work will look at increasing the scope and number of participants and conducting associated analysis to understand dependence among the influencing factors and differences among individuals. In addition, research to understand perceptions of healthcare providers, who also play an important role in the implementation of the PCEHR system, will be pursued in the future as well.

Acknowledgement

This chapter is developed from the author's previous works: "Exploring Individuals' Perceptions on Personally Controlled Electronic Health Record System", *Proceedings of 16th International Conference on Smart Homes, Assistive Technology and Health Telematics*, Singapore, 2018, pp. 285-291.

References

Australian Government (2012), "Personally Controlled Electronic Health Records Act 2012", available at: https://www.legislation.gov.au/Details/C2012A00063, (accessed 14 December 2014).

Australian Taxation Office (2015), "Flood levy", available at: https://www.ato.gov.au/Individuals/Dealing-with-disasters/Previous-years/Flood-levy/Flood-levy/ (accessed 14 July 2016).

Brettel, M., Friederichsen, N., Keller, M. and Rosenberg, M. (2014), "How Virtualization, Decentralization and Network Building Change the Manufacturing Landscape: An Industry 4.0 Perspective", International Journal of Mechanical, Aerospace, Industrial, Mechatronic and Manufacturing Engineering, Vol. 8 No. 1, pp. 37-44.

Consumers Health Forum of Australia (2011), "e-Health and Electronic Health Records: Current Consumer Research, January 2011", available at: https://www.chf.org.au/pdfs/rep/rep-691-eHealthresearch-feb11.pdf (accessed 14 August 2012).

Department of Health (2016), "My Health Record", available at: http://health.gov.au/internet/main/publishing.nsf/Content/ehealth-record (accessed 21 June 2016).

Gao, X., Xu, J., Sorwar, S. and Croll, P. (2013), "Implementation of E-Health Record Systems and E-Medical Record Systems in China", The International Technology Management Review, Vol. 3 No. 2, pp.127-139

Gubbi, J., Buyya, R., Marusic, S. and Palaniswami, M. (2013), "Internet of Things (IoT): A vision, architectural elements, and future directions", Future Generation Computer Systems, Vol. 29, pp.1645-1660.

Kerlin, J. and Heath, J. (2014), "E-health scheme to be revived after panel review", The Australian Financial Review, May 24 2014, Online Available at: http://www.afr.com/business/health/pharmaceuticals/ehealth-scheme-to-be-revived-after-panel-review-20140523-iupi8 (accessed on February 18, 2016).

Review Panel (2014), "Review of the Personally Controlled Electronic Health Record", available at: http://www.health.gov.au/internet/main/publishing.nsf/Content/PCEHR-Review (accessed 14 December 2014).

Sligo, J., Gauld, R., Roberts, V. and Villa, L. (2017), "A literature review for large-scale health information system project planning, implementation and evaluation", International Journal of Medical Informatics, Vol. 97, pp.86-97.

Ventola, C.L. (2014), "Mobile Devices and Apps for Health Care Professionals: Uses and Benefits", PubMed Central, Vol. 39, No. 5, pp.356–364.

Xu, J., Gao, X., Sorwar, G. and Croll, P. (2013), "Implementation of E-Health Record Systems in Australia", The International Technology Management Review, Vol. 3 No. 2, pp.127-139.

Xu, J., Gao, X. and Sorwar, G. (2014), "A research model of consumers' adoption and continued use of the Personally Controlled Electronic Health Record (PCEHR) system", International Technology Management Review, Vol. 4, No.4, pp.187-200.

Chapter 5

Factors Influencing Individual's Decision on Adopting and Continually Using Personal Health Record System: An Australian Study

This chapter reports a study testing the model of PCERH system adoption and continued use discussed in Chapter 1. The data were collected via online questionnaire surveys and were analysed via Structural Equation Modelling (SEM) approach. Identified significant factors influencing the decision regarding system adoption include "External Factors & Influences", "Individual Differences", "Perceived Benefits" of the PCEHR system, PCEHR "System Characteristics", "Perceived User Friendliness" and "Voluntariness of Adoption", while "Realized Benefits", "Realized User Friendliness" and "Voluntariness of Continued Use" are significant factors influencing the decision regarding the continued use of the PCEHR system. The outcomes of the research lead to suggestions to assist the Australian Government in the ongoing rollout/implementation of the system.

Keywords: Electronic Health Records, My Health Record, PCEHR, Adoption, Continued Use, Structural Equation Modelling, Australia.

5.1 Introduction

This research applies convenience sampling approach. Staff and students in an Australian university where the authors work, who are eligible for registering with and using the PCEHR system (i.e., registration restricted to Australian Permanent Residents and Australian Citizens only), were invited to take part in the online questionnaire survey, which asks questions about the participants' adoption and use of the PCEHR system. The message of: "This questionnaire is designed for Australian Permanent Residents and Australian Citizens. If you are not one of them, please kindly ignore the invitation to participate in the research." is highlighted on the cover page of the questionnaire. Furthermore, assurance of only eligible users taking part in the survey is done by having a specific eligibility question in the demographic information part of the questionnaire (the first part of the questionnaire) by asking: "Are you an Australian citizen or permanent resident of Australia?"

Two rounds of e-mail invitations to participate in the research were sent to two generic email lists of staff and students. Sending emails to these two email addresses received the approval from the University and was carried out twice (an original one in late October and a follow-up one in early November). The survey questions were developed from literature on innovation diffusion and technology acceptance (Davis, 1986; Rogers, 1995) and previous studies on the PCERH system in Australia (Xu et al., 2012; Xu et al., 2013; Xu et al., 2014). In addition, the researchers sent the online survey invitation to their networks (i.e., people they know outside of the university).

Structural Equation Modelling (SEM) approach is employed to analyse the collected survey data. Compared with conventional analytical techniques, such as multivariate multiple regression analysis, path analysis and factor analysis, Structural Equation Modelling (SEM) have the following advantages (Holmes-Smith 2001): Capability of examining relationships among dependent or (response or outcome or exogenous) variables; Capability of estimating relationships among latent constructs indicated by observed (or explanatory or endogenous) variables; Capability of measuring recursive and non-recursive relationship between constructs; Capability of allocating unequal weightings for the multiple observed variables of a latent construct; and Capability of allowing for correlations among the measurement errors (error co-variances). It can then be said that SEM approach is suitable for this research (i.e., analysing the relations between constructs in the research model).

Having a sizeable sample population for the approach is critical to produce reliable results (Hox and Bechger, 1998). This study adopts the 'case-to-latent variable' ratio approach (i.e., ratio of sample cases to number of variables in the research model), which is a well-established approach accepted by many researchers (Bentler and Chou, 1987; Tanaka, 1987; Kline, 2011; Bagozzi and Yi, 2012) and the suggested 5:1 ratio of sample cases to number of variables in the research model (Bentler and Chou, 1987; Tanaka, 1987) is used to determine the minimum sample size for running the SEM test in this study. Therefore the sample size of 66 in this research is well suited to SEM analysis (i.e., it is greater than the required 40 samples for the 8 composite variables in the adoption model and greater than the required 30 samples for the 6 composite variables in the continued use model).

Application of SEM steps include: model specification, model identification, model estimation, model testing, and model modification (Byrne, 2001; Hair et al., 2010; Schumacker and Lomax, 2010; Kline, 2011; Arbuckle, 2012). This research adheres to these steps whereby a model is specified and identified. Model estimation determines whether the model can achieve satisfactory fit. Where the model fit is poor, a re-specification should be conducted to explore other theoretically justifiable possible changes. Meanwhile the model test consists of two parts: a measurement model and a structural model (Anderson and Gerbing, 1988; Jöreskog, 1993). The measurement model measures the relationships of observed variables (i.e., measurement items) with their underlying constructs (or factors). The structural model examines the casual relations between the constructs.

SEM can be carried out using various computer programs including Amos, SAS/STAT, EQS, LISREL, Mplus, Mx, RAMONA and SEPATH. These computer programs are used by many researchers and deliver well-founded and comparable results (Kline, 2011). The choice of tool is usually decided by the availability and prior familiarity with specific software package (Garson, 2012). This study selects Amos version 21 because of its ability to generate bootstrapped estimates of standard errors and confidence intervals for all parameter estimates, in addition to the availability of both parametric and non-parametric bootstrapping (Arbuckle, 2012; Kline, 2011).

5.2 Results

5.2.1 Demographic information

Of the 110 responses received, only 66 respondents completed all the questions of the questionnaire (especially sections relating to the research model), so these valid 66 responses are used for the study. On a related note, the data on the research model were collected in the same study reported in Chapter 4.

The respondents report varied e-health experience. 53% of the respondents state they don't have any e-health experience, 34.8% having experience of using electronic systems for healthcare supportive services (e.g., online appointment scheduling, checking in via kiosks, claiming expense online), 15.2% having experience of participating in online health programs (e.g., health and fitness through diet and exercise programs), 13.6% having experience of using telemedicine (i.e., enabling doctors and nurses to see and diagnose patients remotely), 9.1% having experience of online treatments and assessments, 18.2% having experience of using health-related phone/tablets apps, 24.2% having experience of using wearable health and fitness tracking technology, 1.5% gaining e-health experience in registering with the PCEHR system, and 1.5% having e-health research experience.

For survey participants, some most important sources to get information about the PCEHR system include (in order): from the media (including TV, website, radio, newspaper, magazine, or other media Channels) (34.8% of the respondents), from other people (e.g., my friends, my family members, colleagues, neighbours or people I met/talked to) (27.3%), from healthcare providers (15.2%), and from promotion materials received from the government or/and its agencies (15.2%). The majority of the survey respondents (68.2%) lack knowledge of the PCEHR system, and they either have no knowledge/understanding of the PCEHR system or don't know much about the system. 74.2% of the respondents have not been involved in the implementation/roll-out of the PCEHR system, and 77.3% are happy to let health care providers (other than their GP) to access (either on a regular basis or case-by-case manner) their medical information in the system (either full access or partial access). Meanwhile only 33.3% of the survey participants believe the PCEHR system will be successful in the future.

Only 10.6% of the respondents have registered with the system (including registering their dependent children) while another 28.8% suggest that they will register with the system in the future. Among those respondents who have registered, 85% have registered for more than 12 months, 2.5% for more than 24 months, and 4.2% for less than 1 month. 71.4% of respondents registered themselves and the remaining 28.6% have registered with the assistance of government agencies or whilst hospitalised. 57.5% have registered for the system online, 14.2% at their GP's practice/clinic, 14.2% at a mobile station/booth, and 14.2% at the place of a health care provider (other than their GP). In addition, the majority (57.1%) of the registered respondents have not used the system at all after their registration with the system (either don't want to use or don't know how to use the system).

5.2.2 Goodness of Fit

Model estimation is a critical step where the model's goodness-of-fit and parameters are assessed to determine how well the model explains the data (Hu and Bentler, 1999; Kline, 2011). Two primary methods of estimating model fit are those involving X^2 goodness-of-fit statistic and fit indexes (Hu and Bentler, 1999). A good fit is obtained when the X2 statistic is non-significant, which by convention is taken to happen for p-value ≥ 0.05 (Bagozzi and Yi, 2012). Meanwhile, it is also widely accepted that the X^2 statistic is sensitive to sample sizes (McQuitty, 2004). As a result, scholars also recommend assessing the normed X^2 (also known as CMIN/DF), which is obtained by dividing the X^2 statistic by the degrees of freedom, in an attempt to make the X^2 statistic less dependent on sample size (Arbuckle, 2012). Values of three (3) or lower for CMIN/DF is considered acceptable (Hair et al., 2010; Kline, 2011).

The second stream of estimating the goodness-of-fit is by using a number of fit indexes. In this study three fit indexes of CFI, GFI and RMSEA, are selected because of their widespread usage and consistent reference in a majority of academic sources (Hu and Bentler, 1999; Byrne, 2001; Tabachnick and Fidell, 2001; Schumacker and Lomax, 2010; Kline, 2011; Bagozzi and Yi, 2012). CFI is an incremental fit index that measures the relative improvement in the fit of the research model over that of a baseline model (Kline, 2011). CFI for a valid model ranges between zero and one, with values higher than 0.90 considered an acceptable fit (Hu and Bentler, 1999; Hair et al., 2010). The GFI is an absolute fit index that estimates the proportion of co-variances in the sample data matrix explained by the model (Kline, 2011). GFI estimates how much the research model fits compared with no model at all and GFI ranges between zero and one, with values higher than 0.90 considered acceptable (Hair et al., 2010; Kline, 2011). Measures of Population Discrepancy – the Root Mean Square Error of Approximation (RMSEA) is scaled as a badness-of-fit index where a value of zero indicates the best fit (Kline, 2011). Browne and Cudeck (1993) and Hair et al. (2010) recommend RMSEA larger than 0.10 to be a poor fit.

Table-1 summarises the measures adopted in this research to estimate model fit, namely the □2 goodness-of-fit statistic and its p score, CMIN/DF, CFI, GFI and RMSEA, and their respective threshold values.

Table-1: Measures for Estimate Model Fit

If χ^2 and *p* values are...	If CMIN/DF value is...	If CFI value is...	If GFI value is...	If RMSEA value is...	The recommended assessment is...
Insignificant ($p >= 0.05$)	<= 3	>= 0.900	>= 0.900	< 0.100	Model is saturated and the fit is perfect
Significant ($p < 0.05$)	> 3	< 0.900	< 0.900	>= 0.100	Model is rejected and diagnostics undertaken to improve model fit

Table-2 present summaries, iterations and results of model estimates for External Factors & Influences. Composite factor after the model estimation process (including required iterations to remove unfit variables) achieves model saturation and perfect model fit. The same process is applied to all fourteen factors of the model. Table-3 and Table-4 lists the variables of composite factors after the model estimation process for adoption decision factors and continued use decision factors.

Table-2: Summary of Measure Model Estimate for External Factors & Influences

External factors & influences (EX)	Variables	Results	Assessment
Hypothesised Model	EX1 EX2 EX3 EX4 EX5 EX6 EX7 EX8 EX9 EX10	$\chi^2_M(35) = 144.342$ $p = 0.000$ (significant) CMIN/DF = 4.124 CFI = 0.547 GFI = 0.691 RMSEA = 0.219	The hypothesised model is rejected based on significant χ^2 statistic.
Iteration 1	EX1 EX2 EX3 EX5 EX8 EX9	$\chi^2_M(9) = 12.385$ $p = 0.192$ (insignificant) CMIN/DF = 1.376 CFI = 0.946 GFI = 0.941 RMSEA = 0.076	EX4, EX6, EX7 and EX10 have very low standardised regression weights in relation with variable EX. In the interest of parsimony, these variables were removed because of low correlation with other variables. The revised model is saturated

			and the fit is perfect.

Table-3: Variables of Composite Factors of Adoption Decision

Factors and Variables	Explanation
External Factors & Influences	
Regulations and Policies (EX1)	The regulations and policies relevant to the PCEHR system (e.g., Healthcare Identifiers Act 2010, Personally Controlled Electronic Health Records Act 2012) are essential to the implementation of the PCEHR system.
ICT Infrastructure Development (EX2)	The deployment of national broadband and investments in e-heath infrastructure by federal and state governments have laid the foundation for the implementation of the PCEHR system.
Mobility (EX3)	The increasing mobility of population from one place to another needs the PCEHR system so I can access my health information anywhere.
Affordability and Accessibility of Internet Services (EX5)	The high Internet penetration in Australia (more than 85%), as a result of good nationwide technology infrastructure and affordability, has made the PCEHR system more appealing.
Unified Approach (EX8)	Australia's multi-tier government system and large private sector has made the implementation of the PCEHR system extremely complex.
Transparency and Communication of The Operations of the PCEHR System (EX9)	Improved transparency and communication regarding the operations of the PCEHR system could have positive impact on the implementation of the system.
Individual Differences	
Involvement (ID1)	My involvement in the deployment of the PCEHR system would encourage the ownership and lead to the acceptance and use of the system.
Experience/Skill (ID2)	My experience/skill in using new systems and new technologies will affect my acceptance and use of the PCEHR system. The more experienced I am, the more likely I would accept and use the system.
Personal Innovativeness (ID3)	If I am innovative and would like to try new things, I would be more likely to accept and use the PCEHR system.
Computer Skills (ID4)	I have sufficient computer skills, I would be more likely to accept and use the PCEHR system.
Attitude (ID5)	If I don't feel comfortable and/or confident to manage and disseminate my health information electronically, I am less likely to accept and use the PCEHR system.
PCEHR System Characteristics	
Trialability (PS1)	I should be able to try out the PCEHR system before I decide to use the system.
Accuracy, Completeness and Currency of the Information (PS2)	Information in the PCEHR system should be accurate, complete, and current.

Access Control (PS3)	I should be able to see all the activities in my PCEHR system accounts.
Accessibility (PS6)	I should be able to access my electronic health records in the PCEHR system anywhere and anytime via different computing devices and channels.
Cross-border/International Integration (PS10)	The PCEHR system should be integrated well with applications and systems of various healthcare providers outside Australia.
Maintenance and Updates (PS11)	The PCEHR system should be maintained and updated regularly.
Delegation (PS12)	The PCEHR system should allow me to delegate the management of my medical information in the system when necessary.
Perceived/Expected Benefits	
Better and New Services (PB2)	The PCEHR system would help create better and new health services.
Efficiency/Productivity (PB3)	The PCEHR system would help enhance the efficiency/productivity of health services.
Quality (PB5)	The PCEHR system would help improve the quality of health services.
Safety (PB6)	The PCEHR system would help improve the safety of health services for Australian consumers.
Time and Cost Reduction (PB7)	The PCEHR system would help reduce time & cost of health services.
Continuity of Health Services (PB8)	The PCEHR system would ensure the continuity of health services for Australian consumers.
Health and Well-Being (PB9)	The PCEHR system would improve my health/well-being.
Saving Lives (PB10)	The PCEHR system would help save lives.
Equitable Access to Health Services (PB11)	The PCEHR system would help provide equitable access to health services.
Continuity of Health Services (PB12)	The PCEHR system would help improve the continuity of health services.
Perceived/Expected User Friendliness	
Simple to Learn and Use (PU1)	The PCEHR system should be simple to learn and use with simple procedures.
Easy to Register (PU2)	The PCEHR system should be easy to register.
Affordable to Learn and Use (PU3)	The PCEHR system should be affordable to learn and use.
Speed (PU4)	It should be fast to get the required information in the PCEHR system.
Subject Norms	
Peer Pressure/Influence (SN1)	Peers have influence on my acceptance and use of the PCEHR system.
Following Early Users' Lead (SN2)	I would follow earlier users' lead in accepting and using the PCEHR system.
Doctor's Recommendation (SN5)	I would accept and use the PCEHR system as a result of the recommendation from my doctors.
Media Influence (SN6)	I would accept and use the PCEHR system as a result of

	the influence from the media.
Voluntariness	
Opt-in Model (VA1)	The current opt-in model would make me feel comfortable to accept and use the PCEHR system.
Opt-out Model (VA2)	The opt-out model would make me feel comfortable to accept and use the PCEHR system.
Mandatory Use (VA3)	I should be required to use the PCEHR system for my health-related matters.
Linking to Benefits (VA4)	Claims of government benefits & rebates should be linked to the PCEHR system.
Benefit Realization (VA5)	I will use the PCEHR system when I see the benefits of using the system.
System Adoption	
Uploading and Storing Information (SA1)	Uploading and storing my medical information into the PCEHR system.
Disseminating and Sharing Information with Healthcare Providers (SA2)	Disseminating and sharing my health/medical information with various healthcare providers.
Linking with Other Government Services (SA4)	Linking the system with other services provided the government.
Better Understanding of Health Conditions (SA6)	Better understanding my health conditions and having better awareness of my health issues/concerns.

Table-4: Variables of Composite Factors of Continued Use Decision

Factors and Variables	Explanation
Facilitating Factors	
Incentives (FF1)	Appropriate incentives (e.g., concessions and deductions) would encourage me to continue my use of the PCEHR system.
Policy Updates (FF3)	Appropriate policy updates regarding the use of PCEHR system would encourage me to continue my use of the PCEHR system.
System Improvements (FF4)	Continuous system improvements (e.g., being easier for registration, accelerating introduction of more planned features (such as pathology and radiology results), being easier to contribute information, and increasing the range of information in the system) would encourage me to continue my use of the PCEHR system.
Encouragement (FF8)	I should be encouraged to make the use of the PCEHR system a part of my life.
Good Governance (FF9)	Good governance model of the PCEHR system would encourage me to continually use the system.
Better Training (FF11)	Better training of using the system should be provided by the government.
Realized Benefits	
Personal Medical Information Management (RP1)	Has helped me better manage my personal medical information (especially electronically).

Efficiency/Productivity (RP3)	Has helped enhance the efficiency/productivity of health services.
Effectiveness (RP4)	Has helped improve the effectiveness of health services.
Safety (RP6)	Has helped improve the safety of health services.
Saving Lives (RP10)	Has helped save lives.
Realized User Friendliness	
Simple to Learn and Use (RU1)	The PCEHR system has demonstrated to be simple to learn and use with simple procedures.
Easy to Register (RU2)	The PCEHR system has demonstrated to be easy to register. .
Affordable to Learn and Use (RU3)	The PCEHR system has demonstrated to be affordable to learn and use with simple procedures.
Speed (RU4)	It has demonstrated to be fast to get the required information in the PCEHR system.
Privacy (RU6)	The PCEHR system has effectively demonstrated to be able to address the privacy concerns associated with using the system by establishing privacy policies and appropriate measures.
Communities (RU10)	I have been provided with the opportunities to network with other users of the PCEHR system (online and offline).
Subject Norms on Continued Use	
Peer Pressure/Influence (SNP1)	Peers have influence on my continued use of the PCEHR system.
Following Early Users' Lead (SNP2)	I would follow earlier users' lead in continued use of the PCEHR system.
Respected People's Influence (SNP4)	I would continually use the PCEHR system as a result of encouragement from respected people.
Media Influence (SNP6)	I would continually use the PCEHR system as a result of the influence from the media.
Voluntariness of Continued Use	
Opt-in Model (VC1)	The current opt-in model would make me feel comfortable to continually use the PCEHR system.
Mandatory Use (VC3)	I should be required to continually use the PCEHR system for my health-related matters.
Linking to Benefits (VC4)	Claims of government benefits & rebates should be continually linked to the PCEHR system.
Benefit Realization (VC5)	I will continually use the PCEHR system when I have realized the benefits of using the system.
Continued Use	
Uploading and Storing Information (SC1)	Uploading and storing my medical information into the PCEHR system.
Disseminating and Sharing Information with Healthcare Providers (SC2)	Disseminating and sharing my health/medical information with various healthcare providers.
Disseminating and Sharing Information with Government Agencies (SC3)	Disseminating and sharing my health/medical information with government agencies.
Managing Health Information (SC5)	Using the system to manage my health/medical information.

5.2.3 Validity and Reliability of Composite Factors

Before the structural model testing, validity and reliability of composite factors need to be examined. Fourteen composite variables are constructed by taking the mean of interval questions relating to the research model. Table-5 presents the results of validity and reliability of the 14 composite variables.

Validity relates to the ability of an instrument to accurately measure what it was designed to measure and the integrity in which constructs are generated (Davis and Cosenza, 1993; Zikmund, 2003; Manning and Munro, 2007). Developed by Karl Pearson in 1901, Principal Component Analysis (PCA) is one of the most common statistical techniques to reduce a large number of variables to fewer dimensions, called 'principal components' (Holland, 2008; Dwinnell, 2010; UCLA SCG, 2011). The objective of PCA is to condense a set of original variables into a reduced number of factors with a minimal loss of information (Hair et al., 2010). Summative scales and composite variables are often affirmed by using PCA to establish an empirical estimate of the structure of the variables considered (Hair et al., 2010). Manning and Munro (2007) recommend that components with an eigenvalue greater than 1.0 can be considered to be internally valid. The results of PCA are presented in Table-5, which consistently shows a single component extracted for each group of survey items with eigenvalues well above 1.0. These results confirm that the fourteen composite factors are internally consistent and valid.

Reliability is the consistency of a respondent's answer. Reliability is described by Zikmund (2003) as the degree to which survey items are free from error and yield consistent results. Reliability is concerned with the ability of an instrument to measure consistently (Tavakol and Dennick, 2011). The most frequently reported reliability index is Cronbach's coefficient alpha which is the method chosen to affirm reliability in this study (Cronbach, 1951; Iacobucci and Duhachek, 2003; Hair et al., 2008; Tavakol and Dennick, 2011). Cronbach (1951, p.331) defined α as 'the value expected when two random samples of items from a pool are correlated' and that it is 'an index of common factor concentration' which can be used to indicate homogeneity. α scores above 0.70 are commonly acceptable to indicate the reliability of a research instrument (Nunnally, 1978; Iacobucci and Duhachek, 2003; Hair et al., 2008; Tavakol and Dennick, 2011). The α scores for fourteen composite variables are provided in Table-5. As Table-5 suggests that all α scores, except Voluntary adoption (0.576) and Voluntariness on continued use (0.647), are above 0.70. Voluntary adoption and Voluntariness on continued use are accepted for reasons of good validity and have been supported by the literature and past studies as discussed in the previous hypothesis development section. Such results indicate that those composite variables have good reliability.

Table-5: Validity and Reliability of Composite Factors

Composite Factor	Principal Components for Validity		Cronbach's Alpha for Reliability
	Total	% of Variance	
External factors & influences (EX)	2.518	41.966	0.708
Individual factors (ID)	2.600	51.990	0.711
System characteristics (PS)	3.513	50.186	0.813
Perceived benefits (PB)	7.375	73.755	0.960
Perceived user friendliness (PU)	3.063	76.578	0.896
Subject norms (SA)	2.708	67.699	0.837
Voluntary adoption (VA)	1.883	37.656	0.576
System adoption (SA)	2.463	61.575	0.783
Facilitating factors (FF)	3.596	59.931	0.865
Realised benefits (RP)	4.425	88.493	0.967
Realised user friendliness (RU)	4.611	76.851	0.928
Subject norms on continued use (SNP)	2.934	73.340	0.878
Voluntariness on continued use (VC)	1.971	49.271	0.647
Continued use (SC)	2.798	69.939	0.847

5.2.4 Structural Model for Adoption

Table-6 reports the results of the structural model test of adoption of the PCEHR system. The output are assessed based on estimated path coefficient value (β) with critical ratio (t) and probability (p). The absolute value of $t \geq 1.645$ and $p \leq 0.05$ are the thresholds used to accept the hypothesised relationships between the variables (Byrne, 2001; Hair et al., 2010). Furthermore, β evaluates the relative influence of the predicting variable on the dependent variable (Arbuckle, 2012).

For example, when Perceived Benefits increase by 1.0 standard deviation, Adoption Decision is estimated to increase by 0.693 standard deviation.

Table-6 SEM Output for Hypothesised Path Relationships in Structural Model for Adoption Decision

Hypothesis	**Path**	**Standardised Estimate (β)**	**Standard Error (S.E.)**	**Critical Ratio (t)**	**Probability (*p*)**	**Result**
H1(a)	EX → PB	0.387	0.139	2.788	0.005	Supported
H1(b)	EX → PU	0.357	0.161	2.220	0.026	Supported
H2(a)	ID → PB	0.484	0.198	2.447	0.014	Supported
H2(b)	ID → PU	0.585	0.266	2.198	0.028	Supported
H3(a)	PS → PB	0.028	0.064	0.435	0.663	Not Supported
H3(b)	PS → PU	0.778	0.211	3.687	< 0.001	Supported
H4	PU → PB	-0.020	0.170	-0.120	0.905	Not Supported
H5	PB → SA	0.693	0.100	6.944	< 0.001	Supported
H6	PU → SA	0.447	0.150	2.979	0.003	Supported
H7	SN → SA	0.287	0.188	1.524	0.127	Not Supported
H8	VA → SA	0.339	0.133	2.546	0.011	Supported

5.2.5 Structural Model for Continued Use

Table-7 reports the results of the structural model test of continued use of the PCEHR system. Again the output are assessed based on estimated path coefficient value (β) with critical ratio (t) and probability (p). The absolute value of $t \geq 1.645$ and $p \leq 0.05$ are the thresholds used to accept the hypothesised relationships between the variables (Byrne, 2001; Hair et al., 2010). Further, β evaluates the relative influence of the predicting variable on the dependent variable (Arbuckle,

2012). For example, when Realised Benefits increase by 1.0 standard deviation, Continued Use is estimated to increase by 0.601 standard deviation.

Table-7 SEM Output for Hypothesised Path Relationships in Structural Model for Continued Use

Hypothesis	**Path**	**Standardised Estimate (β)**	**Standard Error (S.E.)**	**Critical Ratio (t)**	**Probability (*p*)**	**Result**
H9(a)	FF ➔ RP	0.293	0.141	2.073	0.038	Supported
H9(b)	FF ➔ RU	0.311	0.118	2.630	0.009	Supported
H10	RU ➔ RP	0.489	0.125	3.924	< 0.001	Supported
H11	RP ➔ SC	0.601	0.097	6.226	< 0.001	Supported
H12	RU ➔ SC	0.626	0.120	5.207	< 0.001	Supported
H13	SNP ➔ SC	0.272	0.171	1.586	0.113	Not Supported
H14	VC ➔ SC	0.362	0.115	3.157	0.002	Supported

5.3 Results Discussion

5.3.1 The Adoption Model

The results (as shown in Table-6) indicate that (1) "External Factors & Influences" and "Individual Differences" are significant factors that influence "Perceived Benefits" of the PCEHR system, which in turn influence adoption of the PCEHR system; (2) "External Factors & Influences", "Individual Differences", and "PCEHR System Characteristics" are significant factors that influence "Perceived User Friendliness" of the PCEHR system, which in turn influence adoption of the PCEHR system; and (3) "Voluntariness of Adoption" is a significant factor that influences adoption of the PCEHR system. Meanwhile it is observed that not all the hypotheses are supported. H3a, H4, and H7 are not supported.

H3a-System Characteristics and Perceived Benefits

The result of the non-significant influence of the PCEHR system characteristics on perceived benefits of the PCEHR system, indicates that while the users of the PCEHR system value the system characteristics (e.g., data accuracy, completeness, and currency, accessibility, availability, and information control), their attitude toward (or perceptions of) the system will not be influenced by these characteristics. Some possible reasons include: (1) their lack of engagement/involvement in the PCEHR system rollout/implementation (i.e., 74% respondents), (2) their lack of knowledge of the system (i.e., 68.2% respondents), (3) their lack of e-health experience (i.e., 53% respondents having no e-health experience), (4) low registration/adoption and use of the system (e.g., only 10.6% participants have registered for the system, and the majority (57.1%) of the registered users have not used the system at all after registration), and (5) the users' key concerns are security and privacy concerns which are not covered/addressed by system features (but by system user friendliness factor).

H4-Perceived User Friendliness and

The proposed positive influence of user-friendliness on usefulness of the PCEHR system is not supported by the survey data. One possible explanation is that the usefulness of the PCEHR system is a more important determinant of adoption decision of the system. Users will not adopt the system until they can clearly see the benefits of the system. Furthermore respondents could view the use of the system as extra burden/work for them, which may (or may not) be necessary unless they can clearly realize the benefits of using the system (e.g., better and new health services, better management of their medical information, improving effectiveness and efficiency of health service systems, saving time and money). It is only when respondents see realized benefits, then they will accept and use the system. In addition, as mentioned earlier, as a result of their lack of knowledge of the PCEHR system and engagement/involvement in the roll-out/implementation of the system, and low registration and use of the system, their understanding and experience of the system (including user friendliness of the system) is very limited as well.

H7-Subject Norms and Adoption of the System

It is seen from the results that Subject Norms don't influence users' adoption decision of the PCEHR system. This insignificant relationship is a surprise as past research (Thompson et al., 1991; Lucas and Spitler 1999) has found that Subject Norms are positively associated with the individual's acceptance of new technology, and past studies (Hartwick and Barki, 1994; Taylor and Todd, 1995) have suggested that Subject Norms are more important in early stages of innovation implementation, when users have limited direct experience from which to develop attitudes and perceptions.

A possible explanation is that users/consumers will be more willing to accept and use the system when the use of the system is on the voluntary basis (e.g., opt-in approach) even though Subject Norms (e.g., influence from doctors and respected people) could have an impact on their acceptance and use of the system. On a related note, while trusted people could influence users' decision of accepting and using the system, other issues such as benefits of the system, privacy and security concerns, could have negative impacts on their willingness to try and adopt the system.

In addition, even though users may view the system as being useful and/or user-friendly, they may not be confident enough to use the system themselves for reasons such as lack of knowledge and experience of e-health and the PCEHR system, lack of engagement/involvement in the implementation/roll-out of the system, low registration and use of the system, and they may want their doctors or/and health care providers to manage their health/medical information.

5.3.2 The Continued Use Model

The results (as shown in Table-7) indicate that (1) "Facilitating Factors" are significant factors that influence both "Realized Benefits" and "Realized User Friendliness", which in turn influence continued use of the PCEHR system; and (2) "Voluntariness of Continued Use" is a significant factor that influences continued use of the PCEHR system. Meanwhile it can be seen that H13 is supported.

H13-Subject Norms and Continued Use of the System

The results indicate that Subject Norms don't influence users' continued use of the PCEHR system. It can be argued that even though users may realize the benefits of using the system and may like the functions of the system (as reasons mentioned in the previous discussion of the non-significant influence of Subject Norms on adoption of the PCEHR system), users could still like/want their doctors and/or their health care providers to continually manage their medical/health information on their behalf.

5.4 Discussion

Key findings of the research

Even though the Australian Government has invested significantly in deploying the PCEHR system and its associated infrastructure (including required technological infrastructure, standards, and legislation), the system has not been well accepted by individuals. In addition, there is a lack of comprehensive empirical studies of the current status and challenges/issues as well as reasons and factors for success and/or failure of electronic health record systems, especially the PCEHR system. This research tested a model of adoption and continued use of the PCEHR system and surveyed consumers/users in Australia. The model is unique in the sense that it includes both adoption and continued use of the PCEHR system in one model and many factors and variables are very specific to the PCEHR system adoption and continued use. The collected data were analysed using a structural equation modelling (SEM) approach. The results suggest that, with only a few exceptions, most of the factors of the model are important determinants of users'/consumers' decision of adoption and continued use of the system. Significant factors for adoption of the PCEHR system include: External Factors and Influences, Individual Differences, PCEHR System Characteristics, Perceived Benefits, Perceived User Friendliness, and Voluntariness. Significant factors for continued use include Facilitating Factors, Realized Benefits, Realized User Friendliness, and Voluntariness.

Contribution to the literature and Implications for the practice

This research tested a model of adoption and continued use of the PCEHR system and surveyed consumers/users in Australia. The model is unique in the sense that it includes both adoption and continued use of the PCEHR system in one model and many factors and variables are very specific to the PCEHR system adoption and continued use. The results suggest that, with only a few exceptions, most of the factors of the model (e.g., External Factors and Influences, Individual Differences, System Characteristics, Benefits, User Friendliness, Voluntariness, and Facilitating Factors) are important determinates of users'/consumers' decisions of adoption and continued use of the PCEHR system. Such results are in line with the literature (as discussed in the previous Theoretical Models and Hypotheses section in the paper) and confirm the significance of those factors in influencing the users' decision of adoption and use of the system. As far as the researchers are aware, the tested model of adoption and continued use of the

PCEHR system will be the first one focusing on implementation of the PCEHR system in Australia. The model could be easily adapted for studying other countries' national electronic health record system implementations and the adoption and continued use of other technological applications.

The outcomes from this research can assist in understanding the current status and challenges/issues and the provision of practical guidelines necessary for the successful implementation of the PCEHR system. Identified factors and variables of the model presented in Table-3 and Table-4 can assist in understanding challenges and issues associated with the continuous development and implementation of the system and serve as guidelines to the successful implementation of the system. In addition, the outcomes of this research can make contributions to improve awareness of the system among Australian consumers (e.g., via some most important sources they use to get information about the PCEHR system identified in this research, namely from the media (including TV, website, radio, newspaper, magazine, or other media Channels) (34.8% of the respondents), from other people (e.g., my friends, my family members, colleagues, neighbours or people I met/talked to) (27.3%), from healthcare providers (15.2%), and from promotion materials received from the government or/and its agencies (15.2%)). Furthermore, the results of the project and future projects build on this project will make contribution in achieving economic benefits (such as reduced time for and better accuracy of dealing with health issues of cross-board patients, more competent health work force), environmental benefits (such as reduced time for and better accuracy of accessing and understanding patients, better quality of information of patients, and reduced cost for holding and accessing information per patient), and social benefits (such as happier, more satisfied and more comfortable Australian public).

5.5 Summary

A model of adoption and continued use of the PCEHR system was tested via surveying consumers/individual users in Australia. The model is unique in the sense that it includes both adoption and continued use of the PCEHR system in one model and examines the many factors and variables very specific to the PCEHR system adoption and continued use. The results suggest that with only a few exceptions, most of the factors of the model are important determinants of users'/consumers' decision of adoption and continued use of the PCEHR system.

An obvious limitation of the research is the small sample size. Although the invitation to participation was sent twice via email, which could reach thousands of the staff and students that were eligible to use the system, the participation rate is low since we were not permitted to send individual invitations as per the University's policy but rather only permitted to send blanket invitations via two generic email addresses (i.e., one to all staff in the University and the other to all students in the University). One reason for the low participation rate could be that likely respondents knew very little about the PCEHR system and possibly believed they could add little to the survey which may have included many responses of 'not applicable.' The immediate next step is to test the model using large scale studies (e.g., a national survey of consumers in Australia). Future research could focus on a certain part of the model or extend the model to include more factors and variables not included in this research to understand other topics regarding e-health, which is a much broader topic than just the PCEHR system. Future research could also look at developing and testing a model of adoption and continued use of the PCEHR system among health services providers.

Acknowledgement

This chapter is developed from the author's previous works: "Testing a Model of Adoption and Continued Use of Personally Controlled Electronic Health Record (PCEHR) System Among Australian Consumers: A Preliminary Study", *Proceedings of 16th International Conference on Smart Homes, Assistive Technology and Health Telematics, Singapore*, 2018, pp.121-133.

References

Anderson, J.C. and Gerbing, D.W. (1988), "Structural equation modelling in practice: A review and recommended two-stepped approach", Psychological Bulletin, Vol. 103, No. 3, pp. 411-423.

Arbuckle, J. 2012. Amos 21 User's Guide, IBM.

Bagozzi, R. P. and Yi, Y. (2012), "Specification, evaluation, and interpretation of structural equation models", Journal of the Academy of Marketing Science, Vol. 40, No. 1, pp. 8-34.

Bentler, P. M. and Chou, C. P. (1987), "Practical issues in Structural Modelling", Sociological Methods & Research, Vol. 16, No. 1, pp.78-117.

Browne, M. W. and Cudeck, R. (1993), "Alternative ways of assessing model fit", In: Bollen, K. A. and Long, J. S. (eds.) Testing structural equation models, Newbury Park, CA: Sage.

Byrne, B. M. (2001), Structural Equation Modeling With Amos: Basic Concepts, Applications, and Programming, New York, NY, Lawrence Erlbaum Associates.Carmines, E. G. and McIver, J. P. (1981), "Analyzing models with unobserved variables", In: Bohrnstedt, G. W. and Borgatta, E. F. (eds.) Social measurement: Current issues. Beverly Hills, CA: Sage Publications.

Cronbach, L. J. (1951), "Coefficient Alpha and the Internal Structure of Tests", Psychometrika, Vol. 16, No. 3, pp. 297-333.

Davis, F. D. (1986), A technology Acceptance Model for Empirically Testing New End-User Information Systems: Theory and Results, Doctoral Dissertation, Massachusetts Institute of Technology.

Davis, D. and Cosenza, R. M. (1993), Business research for decision making, Belmont, CA, Wadsworth.

Dwinnell, W. (2010), Principal Components Analysis. Available: http://matlabdatamining.blogspot.com.au/2010/02/principal-components-analysis.html [Accessed 8 July 2014].

Garson, D.G (2012), "Structural Equation Modeling. Statistical Associates Publishing, Asheboro.

Hair, J. F., Black, W., Babin, B. and Anderson, R. (2010), Multivariate data analysis, Upper Saddle River, NJ, Prentice Hall Inc.

Hair, J. F., Bush, R. and Ortinau, D. (2008), Marketing Research, McGraw-Hill Companies Incorporated.

Hartwick, J. and Barki, H. (1994), "Explaining the role of user participation in information system use', Management Science, Vol. 40, No. 4, pp. 440-465.

Holland, S. M. (2008), Principal Components Analysis (PCA), Athens, GA: University of Georgia.

Holmes-Smith, P. (2001), Introduction to Structural Equation Modelling Using LISREL: ACSPRI 2001, Winter Program, School Research, Evaluation and Measurement Services.

Hong, W.Y., Thong, J. Y. L., Wong, W.W. and Tam, K. Y. (2002), "Determinants of user acceptance of digital libraries: an empirical examination of individual differences and system characteristics", Journal of Management Information Systems, Vol. 18, No. 3, pp. 97-124.

Hoque, R. & Sorwar, G. (2017), "Understanding factors influencing the adoption of mHealth by the elderly: An extension of the UTAUT model", International Journal of Medical Informatics, Vol. 101, pp.75-84.

Hox, J. J. and Bechger, T. M. (1998), "An Introduction to Structural Equation Modeling", Family Science Review, Vol. 11, pp. 354-373.

Hu, L. and Bentler, P. M. (1999), "Cutoff criteria for fit indexes in covariance structure analysis: Conventional criteria versus new alternatives", Structural Equation Modeling, Vol. 6, No. 1, pp. 1-55.

Iacobucci, D. and Duhachek, A. (2003), "Advancing Alpha: Measuring Reliability with Confidence", Journal of Consumer Psychology, Vol. 13, No. 4, pp. 478-487.

Jöreskog, K.G. (1993), "Testing structural equation models", in Testing Structural Equation Models, eds K.A. Bollen, and J.S. Long , SAGE Publications, Newbury Park, California, USA, pp. 294-316.

Kline, R. B. (2011), Principles and practice of structural equation modeling, New York, NY, The Guilford Press.

Lucas, H. C. and Spitler, V. K. (1999), "Technology use and performance: a field study of broker workstations", Decision Sciences, Vol. 30, No. 2, pp. 291-311.

Manning, M. and Munro, D. (2007), The Survey Researcher's SPSS Cookbook, Sydney, NSW, Pearson Education Australia.

McQuitty, S. (2004), "Statistical power and structural equation models in business research", Journal of Business Research, Vol. 57. No. 2, pp.175–183.

Nunnally, J. C. (1978), Psychometric Theory, New York, NY, McGraw-Hill.

Rogers, E. M. (1995), Diffusion of Innovations, Fourth Edition, The Free Press, New York, USA.

Schumacker, R. E. and Lomax, R. G. (2010), A Beginner's Guide to Structural Equation Modeling, New York, NY, Routledge.

Tabachnick, B. G. and Fidell, L. S. (2001), Using multivariate statistics, Boston, MA, Allyn and Bacon.

Tanaka, J.S. (1987), "How big is big enough: Sample size and Goodness of Fit in Structural Equation Models with Latent Variables", Child Development, Vol. 58, pp.134-146.

Tavakol, M. and Dennick, R. (2011), "Making sense of Cronbach's alpha", International Journal of Medical Education, Vol. 2, pp. 53-55.

Taylor, S. and Todd, P .A. (1995), "Understanding information technology usage: a test of competing models", Information Systems Research, Vol. 6, No. 2, pp. 145-177.

Thompson, R. L., Higgins, C. A. and Howell, J. M. (1991), "Personal computing: toward a conceptual model of utilization", MIS Quarterly, Vol. 15, No. 1, pp. 125-143.

Thurston, J. (2014), "Meaningful use of Electronic Health Records", The Journal of Nursing Practitioners, Vol. 10, Issue 7, pp. 510-513.

UCLA SCG. (2011), Principal Components Analysis, Los Angeles, CA: UCLA Academic Technology Services. Online, Available: http://www.ats.ucla.edu/stat/SPSS/output/principal_components.htm [Accessed on 8 July 2014].

Xu, J., Gao, X., and Sorwar, G. (2014), "A research model of consumers' adoption and continued use of the Personally Controlled Electronic Health Record (PCEHR) system", International Technology Management Review, Vol. 4, No.4, pp. 187-200.

Xu, J., Gao, X., Sorwar, G. and Croll, P. (2012), "Current Status, Challenges, and Outlook of E-Health Record Systems in Australia", 7th International Conference on Intelligence Systems and Knowledge Engineering, Dec 15-17, 2012, Beijing, China.

Xu, J., Gao, X., Sorwar, G. and Croll, P. (2013), "Implementation of E-Health Record Systems in Australia", International Technology Management Review, Vol. 3, No.2, pp. 92-104.

Zikmund, W. G. (2003), Business Research Methods, Mason, OH, South-Western, Cengage.

Zmud, R. W. (1979), "Individual differences and MIS success: a review of the empirical literature", Management Science, Vol. 25, No. 10, pp. 966-979.

Made in the USA
Monee, IL
04 November 2026

67386116R10061